Angelic Lifestyle

For anyone wishing to have and keep their body in perfect attunement

A Vibrant Lifestyle
from Grand Reiki Master,
Constance Santego

BOOKS CONSTANCE HAS WRITTEN

"The Intuitive Life, A Guide to Self Knowledge
and Healing through Psychic Development"

"Fairy Tales, Dreams and Reality…
Where are you on your path?"

"Your Persona… the Mask You Wear
Understanding your personality traits.
What is your personality and why does it matter?"

Copyright © 2017 Constance Santego
All rights reserved. No part of this book shall be reproduced, stored in a retrieval system or transmitted by any means, electronic, mechanical, photocopying, recording or otherwise, without permission from the publisher. No patent liability is assumed with respect to the use of the information contained herein. Although every precaution has been taken in the preparation of this book, the publisher and author assume no responsibility for errors or omissions. Neither is any liability assumed for damages resulting from the use of information contained herein.
The author and publisher specifically disclaim any responsibility for any liability, loss or risk, personal or otherwise, which is incurred as a consequence, directly or indirectly, of any use and application of any of the contents of this book.

Published by Thoughtweft Publishing Inc.
Kelowna, BC

Cover art: Amy Enoch
Interior/exterior design and copy edit: Stephen Ikesaka

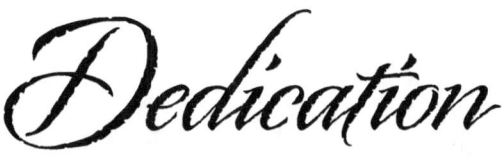

To Reiki, Bill Blaine and
the opportunity to help others create a vibrant lifestyle

Table of Contents

Acknowledgements	9
Preface	11
Angelic Lifestyle	17
Heavenly Day	21
Angelic Foods Shopping List	23
Angelic Foods Meal Plan	30
Fast Food Restaurants	41
Popcorn	44
Rice	45
For Your Wellbeing	47
~ Anatomy/Physiology of the Nervous System	49
~ Memory	55
~ Limbic System	56
~ The Mind	60
~ Anatomy/Physiology of the Digestive System and Nutrition	62
~ Does Death begin in the Colon? Take the test to find out	72
Detoxification	87
Tests to Take	96
Nutritional Facts	101
For Your Health	113
~ Sugar / Diabetes Diet Suggestion	1115
~ Cholesterol / Heart Attack Diet Suggestion	117
Ketosis	119
Natural Health Techniques	123
~ What is Muscle Testing?	124
~ Chinese Body Clock	126
~ Other Types of Sessions that will Benefit your Body	129
Your Emotions and Eating	139
~ Organs and Emotional meaning	141
Emotional Clearing	143
~ Meditation	145
What is your Carrot?	149
~Meditation session #2	152
What if I Fail?	155
The Important Role of Fitness	163
~ Some forms of exercise	166

~ Eight Essential Standing Exercises	170
~ Easy exercises to develop your core	173
~ Walking	178
~ Yoga	179
Glossary	181
Bibliography	185
About the Author	187

Acknowledgements

I would like to thank my friends and family, Alicia Brummet, Kimerley Ellis, Linda Henry, Tracy Fletcher and Tricia Stetar for helping me write this book.

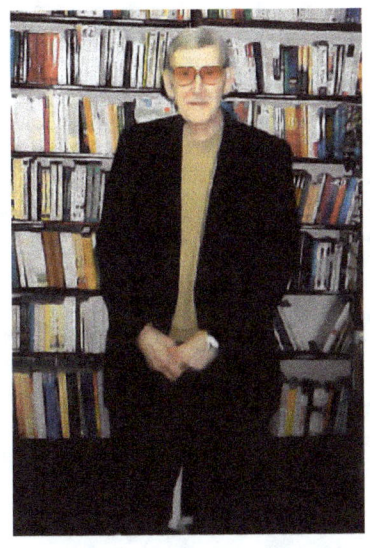

I would like to give a very special thank you to the late Bill Blaine, for four years we shared an office space. He owned a Natural Health book and vitamin business, which I bought off him when he retired. He retired, yes retired, at the age of 95. I remember thinking, will he remember tomorrow? He did.

Bill was a God send and a great mentor! He changed my belief on what old people were; old, unfit, diminishing vitality and losing their minds. He was none of those things. I loved working with him.

He told me he became a vegetarian at the age of fifty. He was in the military, smoked, and drank a little. His first wife had passed away, and he later married a seventh day Adventist lady, who was a vegetarian. He said he just ate more cheese and eggs. After a few years, he had to go to the United States and have Chelation Therapy (Chelation Therapy is a safe, effective, non-surgical treatment used to prevent and treat hardening of the arteries and other degenerative illnesses), due to all the cholesterol build-up. He had to go to the USA because it was not offered in Canada at that time. That is when he became a vegan (well, he never said he was a vegan because he liked his honey – bees have eyes), but he was one to me.

He would study health books, and then follow what he learnt. First thing in the morning he would eat two pieces of Squirrelly, Silver Hills sprouted grain bread covered with tahini (sesame seed spread). For lunch, he would eat one type of fruit (grapes, tomato, or avocado) and nuts – two Brazil nuts and eight almonds. For supper, he would eat steamed vegetables (he said raw vegetables were too hard to digest at his age). He ate like this every day.

You should have seen his living room... I mean fitness room. He loved his rebounder!

One day after he had retired, he came by to say hello and picked up his monthly cheque (for buying his books from him), and he told me he was starting to lose his memory. He seemed to be forgetting what day of the week it was. When he came in the next time, he said that he started to eat chicken and wild salmon (only wild though!) to regain his memory. It worked, and shortly after introduction of these two proteins into his daily diet his memory improved.

When I would ask him a question on what I should do for my health, he would always go pick out some books for me and say read! So, I did. I read and read, and am still reading to this day about health.

Bill, thank you for all that you shared with me, I know I am not the only one that misses you!!!

Preface

To all who know me as Connie

Back in 2010 I was teaching a Reiki class, and just before the initiation a thought popped in my head (or some may say it was a voice). It told me to join in. I was a little taken back, since I had taught this class for many years and never had this idea cross my mind.
So, I decided to listen and I participated. At the end of the initiation I had the class write down any thoughts or messages they had, and I did the same. I had been told that I was just initiated into Grand Reiki Mastery, and that I was required to fulfil the list I had just written down from my meditated state.

There were probably about twenty things I was required to do. That day, I started to tackle my list and fulfil the requirements to become a Grand Reiki Master. One of the requirements was to create and retain a healthy lifestyle for ten months. It seemed simple enough, and I created what I now call Angelic foods.

The assignment of eating Angelic Foods lasted 282 days, with only one day each 42 days (which I called a Heavenly Day) that I could eat anything I wanted all day long. I remember people asking me how I felt while on this assignment. I would tell them that I was tempted to cheat every day, but my "carrot" was big enough to give up anything! In this case my carrot was the title, "Grand Reiki Master", and I wanted that more than the bread, pasta and goodies.

After the assignment was over, and I was not tied to losing the title of being called Grand Reiki Master, I went back to my old eating habits. It did not take much time before I could easily tell the difference between the good feeling of Angelic foods and the bad feeling of reverting back to old eating habits.

In my mind I didn't actually become a Grand Reiki Master until 2016… for two reasons.

1. I didn't do one of the requirements asked of me back in 2010, which was to sell my school to my daughter. (In hindsight I sure wish I had)
2. I did not teach Reiki again until 2016

This was the day I knew I wanted, and needed, to change forever. Not just because of a title, but because I was so tired of all these feelings:
- My clothes didn't fit properly
- My bra got so tight that it was hard to breath
- I would get the shakes from not eating on time
- I would swell just before I had to go pee, and it was a lot harder to wipe my bottom
- I got flushed when I did a lot of physical work
- I had a hard time breathing when I walked up stairs or long distances
- I could feel the fat between my thighs
- I could feel my body fat jiggle when I walked
- It was hard to bend over or squat to pick something up
- By supper time, my socks are cutting into my ankles
- My ribs hurt even while sitting
- I was embarrassed for my husband to see me
- And sadly, my wedding rings did not fit anymore

An Example of Body vs Mind

One day, my son brought home a four person chess game. He and I decided to play it by ourselves since we didn't have four players available. The game is set up like the two player version, except the board is bigger and accommodates four players, one on each side of the square board. I played the player in front of me, silver, and the spot directly across from me, gold. He played the other two, white and black.

The game has the same rules and moves as the traditional version, taking turns in a clockwise fashion. All individual pieces can only move in the traditional patterns. The big difference is you have four sets of chess pieces on the board at one time instead of two and you can capture any of the other three players', but if you are only playing with two players then you only want to capture the other person's two colours.

We started the game as usual; the first player moves a game piece. I started the game by moving one of my silver pieces on the board. He moved a black piece, I moved gold, he a white piece, and so forth.

At first there was nothing new to the game, we just kept moving the appropriate coloured piece. After quite a few moves is when the weird stuff started to happen; I had a move that could capture one of his pieces.
He abruptly said "Mom, you can't do that. It's not that colour's turn." He was correct, it wasn't, so I moved the correct coloured piece without capturing and allowed him to take his turn

My next move came and I tried to capture another piece. Again, he said as he shook his head and made a face like I was nuts, "Mom, wrong colour." It took me by surprise that I had just made the same mistake.
I started to write down what colour I was so I wouldn't make the mistake again.

It didn't help! I was still moving the wrong colour when I saw a chance to capture. So I started to say the colour out loud AND write it down... that didn't help either. It took fourteen tries and a lot of weird looks from my son before I started to be able to move the correct coloured piece in its own turn.

After we were done the game... of course he won... I called my husband on his cell phone (he was working a bit late) and told him what had just happened. I asked him to play our son when he got home to see what experience hed have.

After my husband ate his dinner, he and our son started to play the game. I was in the next room watching TV, so I couldn't influence the game at all. My husband already had the heads up of what happened to me and was sure he wasn't going to make the same mistakes.

My husband and I had been playing chess for over twenty years. We knew the rules and were pretty good competitors for each other. Our son had just started playing just a few years before and could already beat us. About fifteen minutes into the game, I heard my husband's first "Sh*t". I smiled, and a few minutes later, another one. I could hear our son saying, "Dad, you're doing what Mom did." My husband started to fidget on his chair.

"Told you it wasn't so easy," I said.

A few minutes later I heard him say, "This is a stupid game." Meaning he was moving the wrong coloured piece out of turn again.

Our son won that game too.

Later, my husband said he would never play it again, and I replied "It's just another game. We will just need to practice and learn it better". He never did play again; I did though.

My son and I played it a couple more times, and each time I was much better. I learned to not make the mistake of moving the wrong coloured piece out of turn, finally.

I still remember how strange it was in the first game; I knew what colour I was, but I got caught up in capturing that I acted on instinct instead. My body just did it even though I was writing it down and saying it out loud.

What a feeling, to be out of control; my mind wanting one thing and my body doing another... having a subconscious reaction from my body. I assume it's the same for eating, sex, spending money, drugs, alcohol, travel, health and so forth... our minds may know what the best thing to do is, but our body (maybe instincts/habits) seem to just do another.

Another Example:
Have you ever moved to a new home or started a new job, and in the first couple of days driving there you somehow ended up driving to the old place? It's your body's instinct, not your conscious mind.

I also learned that 'practice makes (just about) perfect'. Our body is amazing, and if you put your mind to something you can achieve it!
So that's why it's so hard to follow a new way of eating... you need a carrot for the brain to want more than the food. On the Angelic Foods diet YOU are not starving the body, actually you are probably feeding it the best nutrients it has received in years. Following the Angelic Foods diet will create amazing whole body wellness, and most people will lose weight following the rules.

For those of you who need to know the scientific details of how and why your body and mind work either for or against you in a diet change, the following pages will give basic explanations of the digestive and nervous systems. For those of you who get bored with reading scientific details, please at least skim over the pages, because there are some really interesting facts as well as a test you can take to find out how well your digestive system is doing.

Angelic Lifestyle

By Constance Santego

Disclaimer

Please note that you should check with your Doctor before starting any new eating or fitness regimen. The Angelic Lifestyle does suggest that you follow the Canadian Food Guide, with exception to the process of grains. Grains can be eaten flaked, but not ground.

  Reiki practitioners and body workers are not Doctors, and cannot diagnose, prescribe or change medication. Any advice given by a practitioner is solely personal opinion based on life experience and training.

Angelic Lifestyle

The Angelic Lifestyle is so simple that anyone can do it.

All you have to ask yourself is this:

"Does that food come naturally from nature?"
or
"If I cook this food, will heating it up minimally change the nutrients or the chemical makeup?"

If not... you cannot eat it.
If yes... then go ahead. You can eat any combination, any amount, anytime of the day!

<u>Angelic Foods</u> are foods purchased at the supermarket, and are as minimally processed as conveniently possible!

- Any type of meat, including fish and seafood
- Beans and legumes
- Coconut milk, soy milk
- Dairy products such as:
- Milk, cream, sour cream, cheese (including cottage and cream cheese), yogurt, butter and vanilla ice cream (remember, all can be made naturally).
- Eggs
- Fruit
- Herbs and spices
- Nuts
- Rice
- Sugar in natural form; brown sugar, sugar cane or maple syrup
- Tea or coffee
- Vegetables including potatoes
- Water and natural juice (fruit or vegetable)
- Whole grains or flaked grains only

(A double NO, NO; not ground, or made into bread, pasta or noodles)

It is this simple! All the good foods your body needs to live but not what the brain craves.

The Angelic foods lifestyle is not new. In history, our ancestors all ate like this... real foods.

So why shift to this Reiki lifestyle? For your Health, a positive Vibration and for homeostasis.

Hint: When you are at a grocery store, all the natural foods are set up on display around the outside perimeter. The junk, fattening or processed foods are in the center rows.

Special note, about ground grains:
Ground grains were left out due to the fact that there is barely any natural fiber left, and most of the particles can be absorbed into the body too quickly, causing an insulin jump which could kick your system into shock. Flaked grains are okay to eat!

For the first few days of giving up simple carbohydrates, you might have feelings of withdrawal, starvation, headaches and/or nervousness. Just keep drinking water, and decide what your carrot is. Some of you may need to talk to your physician first before starting any new diet.

At our Natural Health Center, our Musclologists first have the client go to the doctor and have their blood tested to make sure there are no other conditions to worry about that may have been throwing their system into chaos.

- Doctor's blood tests
- Naturopath – allergy and hair analysis

Once you know the balance and levels of your sugar, cholesterol and minerals, if you have any allergies, and have the go ahead to start this new eating plan from your doctor, here is what you would do next:
- Learn to Meditate
- Find your carrot in meditation
- Muscle Test your organs
- Make a breakfast, snack, lunch and dinner/supper meal plan
- Go shopping for the food
- Have a Session and Muscle Test how often you should return. (1/week, month, etc.)
    - European Lymph Drainage Massage
    - Foot Reflexology

- Table Shiatsu
- Beauty Tek
- Body wrap
- Meditation
- Yoga, Qi Gong, Tai Chi or join a fitness program
- Have hypnotherapy counselling sessions as needed

Our clients usually start with seeing us three times a week for the first few weeks, then twice per week, once per week, and then once a month.

HEAVENLY DAY

This is one day every forty-two days that you can eat anything you want (as long as you are not allergic to it, or for any other health reasons).

Go ahead and pig out. Have all those goodies that you've been craving, but I will warn you, your mind is going to play tricks on you!

Here's what happens to me:
- I craved pizza before I created the 'rizza' (rice instead of bread bottom), and actually, pizza is the only food that still tastes good on my Heavenly Day.
- Another craving was spaghetti, but since I went to spaghetti squash I have no more craving.
- When I eat chips or nacho chips, the first bites taste weird. Of course, I would force myself to eat them since my mind remembers that they taste good (The cravings lessen the longer you're eating the Angelic Foods way, because you train the mind to notice the difference between what makes you feel good and what makes you feel bloated).
- Candies and chocolate taste funny. Again, I actually had to force myself to eat them because I remembered they were supposed to taste good, not because they did.
- Bread – only fresh bread still tasted good!

Here is the <u>warning</u>. You will gain weight back extremely quickly. I have gained five pounds, and it takes triple the days just to get back to where you were. Not only that, but you will crave the foods again and it may take a lot of willpower to return to the Angelic Foods way. You may find yourself eating crazily for two or three days instead of just one.

Just make sure you get back to your Angelic Foods right away. After a few Heavenly Days, you will maintain more self control as your body becomes accustomed to the wonderful feeling you have when you are on your

Angelic Foods.. If you are having problems getting back to eating the Angelic Foods way, book an Emotional Clearing or Hypnotherapy Session right away!

It's been proven that having a day where you eat anything shocks your body, and when you go back to eating healthy you will lose more inches and eventually more weight, but only once every month and a half.

Later you can time your Heavenly Day to fit with special occasions, such as your birthday, Christmas, Thanksgiving, Easter, etc.

THIS IS NOT A DIET TO LOSE WEIGHT! THIS IS A DIET TO BE HEALTHY
(YOU MIGHT END UP LOSING SOME FAT THOUGH)

Shopping List

Purchase your items week in advance
<u>Do not</u> purchase any items you are allergic to.

Seasonings

HERBS
- Basil
- Bay (cannot eat – just to add flavour)
- Chives
- Cilantro
- Dill
- Fennel
- Marjoram (careful – can nullify emotions and sex drive)
- Mint
- Oregano
- Parsley
- Rosemary
- Sage
- Savory
- Tarragon
- Thyme

SPICES (FRESH, DRIED OR POWDERED)
- Celery seed
- Cinnamon
- Cloves
- Cocoa
- Coriander seed
- Curry powder
- Garlic (great antioxidant)
- Ginger (fresh – makes a great tea)
- Horseradish

- Mustard
- Onion
- Paprika
- Pepper (Black, cayenne or red)
- Poppy seeds
- Salt (sea salt is best)
- Turmeric
- Vanilla

SOY SAUCE
- Braggs is a healthy brand

NATURAL SUGAR – CAREFUL, HIGH IN CALORIES
- Stevia (herbal sweetener) – powdered or liquid (also comes flavored – chocolate, raspberry or vanilla)
- Brown sugar
- Maple syrup
- Sugar cane

VINEGAR (GREAT FOR SALAD DRESSINGS)
- Balsamic vinegar
- Apple cider vinegar (great brand is Braggs)

PRE-MIXED SEASONINGS
- Mrs. Dash
- Cajun seasoning
- Chili seasoning
- Chinese five spice
- Greek

Liquids
(up to eight glasses a day)

WATER – HELPS FLUSH TOXINS
- Helps suppress your appetite
- The larger you are, the more water you should drink

- Add some lemon to it!

Chlorophyll
- Green pigmentation found in plants. (Excellent nutritional value, prevents body odour, mouth and throat inflammation)

Tea
- Green tea (great antioxidant)
- Non-caffeinated; herbal

Coffee
- A natural diuretic – you will need to drink more fresh water if you drink coffee

Natural Juice
- Too much can be bad for your teeth; you could cut it half water.

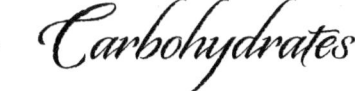

Carbohydrates

Glucose (sugar) turns into glycogen = energy. If you do not use it right away, the excess will be stored in your fat cells for later use.

Complex
Vegetables! The first four items have less calories than it takes to eat them
- Celery
- Cucumber
- Lettuce
- Watercress
- Alfalfa sprouts (great nutritional value)
- Artichokes
- Arugula
- Asparagus
- Avocado (really a fruit)
- Bamboo shoots
- Beans
- Bean sprouts
- Bok choy

- Broccoli (great antioxidant) – Best steamed
- Brussels sprouts – Best steamed
- Cabbage – Best steamed
- Carrots (high in sugar, but also has antioxidants)
- Cauliflower – Best steamed
- Chicory
- Chilli peppers
- Dill pickles
- Eggplant
- Endive
- Green onions
- Kale – Best steamed
- Leeks
- Mushrooms
- Okra
- Olives
- Onions
- Peas
- Peppers (green, red, orange or yellow)
- Radicchio
- Radish
- Rapini
- Snow peas
- Spaghetti squash
- Spinach (antioxidant) – Best steamed
- Swiss chard
- Tomato (really a fruit and a great antioxidant)
- Zucchini

SIMPLE
Turn into sugar quicker
- Whole or flaked grains only! (contains antioxidants)
    - Barley (great in soups)
    - Buckwheat
    - Corn
    - Oat
    - Quinoa
    - Rice or wild rice (brown rice takes longer for the body to turn into sugar)

- Rye
- Wheat (turns to sugar the quickest) Not ground or made into bread, pasta or noodles
- Potatoes

FRUIT
(Most fruit contains traces of antioxidants)
- Apples (rich in antioxidants and two minerals called boron – to keep bones healthy and strong, and pectin – which help prevent cholesterol build up)
- Apricots
- Bananas
- Berries (great antioxidants)
    - Blackberry
    - Blueberry
    - Cranberry
    - Currants
    - Strawberries
    - Saskatoon berries
- Figs
- Grapefruit
- Kiwi
- Cherries
- Grapes (red – antioxidant)
- Lemons
- Limes
- Mango
- Melons
- Honey dew
- Cantaloupe
- Watermelon
- Nectarines
- Oranges
- Peaches
- Pear
- Pineapple
- Dried fruit like raisins, cranberries, cherries

Protein

Burns fat, but too much can cause cholesterol problems.

- Soy milk
- Beans and legumes
    - Black
    - Lima
    - Lentils
    - Pinto
    - Red
    - Red kidney
    - White
- Seeds (Essential fatty acids, omega 3, 6 and 9, reduce the formation of blood clots and promotes strong bones, the production of hormones, energy and absorption of vitamins, metabolism regulation, and healthy cholesterol levels, hair, skin and nails).
- Store in the refrigerator.
    - Flax seed (great source of protein, omega 3 and 6, lignans (have both oestrogenic and anti oestrogenic activity – phytoestrogens).
    - Pumpkin seed (also a great parasite cleanser)
    - Sesame seed
    - Sunflower
- Nuts (best are almonds and brazil nuts; peanuts and cashews have more calories)
    - Peanut butter (best if you grind your own and add a little olive oil)

Dairy Products

- Goat's milk
- Cow's milk (less % = Less calories)
- Yogurt (vanilla only, you can add you own fruit)
- Sour cream
- Cheese (including cottage and cream cheese)
- Butter
- Cream
- Vanilla ice cream (no more than once per week)

Eggs

Meat

In order of calories (try to buy lean – remove any visible fat)
- Fish
    - Cod
    - Halibut
    - Sole
    - Trout
    - Tuna
    - Wild salmon (great for improving your memory)
- Seafood
    - Shrimp/Prawns
    - Octopus
    - Squid (pan fried)
    - Scallops
    - Mussels
    - Oysters
    - Crab
    - Lobster
- Chicken (skinless)
- Turkey
- Lamb
- Wild game – Moose, deer, elk, etc.
- Buffalo
- Beef
    - Steak (fat removed)
    - Extra lean ground beef
    - Any other cut
- Pork
    - Bacon
    - Chops
- Coconut milk (very high in calories)

Fats

Unheated = good fats – needed for energy, production of hormones, conduction of nerve impulses, skin and hair repair, to absorb fat soluble vitamins, mental stability, bowel regulation, and extra fuel, if needed).

VEGETABLE OILS
- Flax seed oil (great for omega 3, 6 and 9 – should be refrigerated)
- Sesame seed oil
- Extra virgin olive oil (refrigerated turns solid, can use as a butter, just mix with some salt first)
- Grapeseed oil

Meal Plan

For the first four weeks, write down what you are eating. If you are eating more often, just write in the times.

WEEK ONE

Date:

	Time	Food eaten	Water
Snack			
Breakfast			
Lunch			
Dinner			

Weight:

Date: _____

	Time	Food eaten	Water
Snack			
Breakfast			
Lunch			
Dinner			

Date: _____

	Time	Food eaten	Water
Snack			
Breakfast			
Lunch			
Dinner			

Date: _____

	Time	Food eaten	Water
Snack			
Breakfast			
Lunch			
Dinner			

Date:

	Time	Food eaten	Water
Snack			
Breakfast			
Lunch			
Dinner			

Date:

	Time	Food eaten	Water
Snack			
Breakfast			
Lunch			
Dinner			

Date:

	Time	Food eaten	Water
Snack			
Breakfast			
Lunch			
Dinner			

Weight:

Week Two

Date:

	Time	Food eaten	Water
Snack			
Breakfast			
Lunch			
Dinner			

Date:

	Time	Food eaten	Water
Snack			
Breakfast			
Lunch			
Dinner			

Date:

	Time	Food eaten	Water
Snack			
Breakfast			
Lunch			
Dinner			

Date:

	Time	Food eaten	Water
Snack			
Breakfast			
Lunch			
Dinner			

Date:

	Time	Food eaten	Water
Snack			
Breakfast			
Lunch			
Dinner			

Date:

	Time	Food eaten	Water
Snack			
Breakfast			
Lunch			
Dinner			

Date:

	Time	Food eaten	Water
Snack			
Breakfast			
Lunch			
Dinner			

Weight:

WEEK THREE

Date:

Time	Food eaten	Water

Snack
Breakfast
Lunch
Dinner

Date:

Time	Food eaten	Water

Snack
Breakfast
Lunch
Dinner

Date:

Time	Food eaten	Water

Snack
Breakfast
Lunch
Dinner

Date:

	Time	Food eaten	Water
Snack			
Breakfast			
Lunch			
Dinner			

Date:

	Time	Food eaten	Water
Snack			
Breakfast			
Lunch			
Dinner			

Date:

	Time	Food eaten	Water
Snack			
Breakfast			
Lunch			
Dinner			

Date:

	Time	Food eaten	Water
Snack			
Breakfast			
Lunch			
Dinner			

Weight:

Week Four

Date:

	Time	Food eaten	Water
Snack			
Breakfast			
Lunch			
Dinner			

Date:

	Time	Food eaten	Water
Snack			
Breakfast			
Lunch			
Dinner			

Date:

	Time	Food eaten	Water
Snack			
Breakfast			
Lunch			
Dinner			

Date:

	Time	Food eaten	Water
Snack			
Breakfast			
Lunch			
Dinner			

Date:

	Time	Food eaten	Water
Snack			
Breakfast			
Lunch			
Dinner			

Date:

	Time	Food eaten	Water
Snack			
Breakfast			
Lunch			
Dinner			

Date:

	Time	Food eaten	Water
Snack			
Breakfast			
Lunch			
Dinner			

Weight:

Fast Food Restaurants

What do you do when you are in a rush and need to eat at a fast food restaurant?

Every once in awhile, you will be in a hurry and need something quick. Remember, in most shopping malls there is a food court that has a lot of healthy choices.

If you can, your first choices should be:
- Japanese
    - Sushi
    - Rice, meat and veggies
- Vietnamese
    - Meat, veggies and rice
- Booster Juice Smoothie
- Salad or Soup

Unfortunately, most Chinese foods are made with batter and deep fried, so keep to rice and some meats. Of course, veggies that have no batter are an option as well.

Next choices, in order:
- If you have to eat a hamburger or breakfast muffin, do not eat the bun!!!
- No French fries. They are deep fried, and the oil turns bad for you when heated to high temperatures.
    - Read the book 'Good Fats Bad Fats: An Indispensable Guide to All the Fats You're Likely to Encounter', by Rosemary Stanton
- Wendy's
    - Any salad (don't eat the croutons or taco chips)
    - Baked potato
    - Chili con carne
- Dairy Queen
    - Vanilla ice cream, plain or with pineapple (the sauce with the least amount of additives)
- All the rest
    - Hot dog, no bun
    - Taco, no shell
    - Chicken, peel the skin coating
    - Pizza, only the topping

If you desperately have to eat and there is no other choice, well, you can't starve! Eat something as healthy as possible, and next time bring a snack.

POPCORN

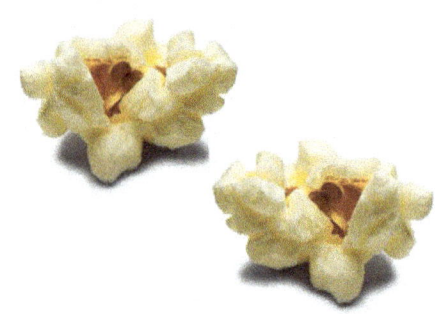

I find it extremely exciting that popcorn is natural and it grows like sweet corn. The only difference is that it is a different kind of kernel that is planted.

The popcorn plant grows and looks similar to other types of corn on the cob. It has a longer growing season (May to Nov), and needs to mature before the first frost. The popcorn plant must turn brown before harvesting, and is harvested in the same process that is used to harvest field corn.

Ever wondered how popcorn pops? Each kernel contains a small amount of water in the middle. As the kernel heats up, the water begins to expand and the pressure inside the kernel builds, causing the soft starch inside the popcorn to explode, almost turning the kernel inside out.

Voila... the popcorn is popped! Popcorn for your Health

Amazingly this little snack is great for preventing cancer, diabetes, heart disease and pancreas issues.

AS QUOTED

The U.S. study was led by Dr. Vinson, a chemist from the University of Scranton in Pennsylvania. He was the first to establish that snack foods, and some wholegrain breakfast cereals, are a good source of polyphenols.

He said, 'We really were surprised by the levels of polyphenols we found in popcorn. I guess it's because it's not processed. You get all the wonderful ingredients of the corn undiluted and protected by the skin. In my opinion it's a good health food.'

RICE

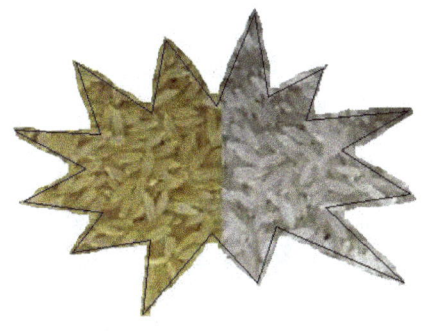

All rice that grows from the earth is brown rice, and is grown in many different countries. The type of rice (long, short, jasmine, wild, etc. – over 40,000 different varieties) will depend on the location, climate and nutrients in the soil.

White rice is produced manually by milling (husking) the brown rice. The outer shell, bran and germ are removed (like a nut being removed from its shell).

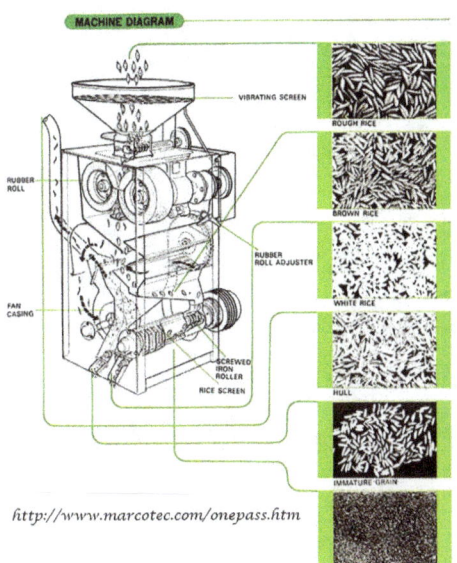

http://www.marcotec.com/onepass.htm

Brown rice is better for you, due to the fact that the body has to work harder to digest the inside (white part). When you eat brown rice, your body will need to get to the inside of the rice to get to the nutrients. The shell is considered fiber (indigestible) and will be eliminated from the body. This means, if you eat only white rice, the work has already been done for you and the body can easily digest all of it, turning it into carbohydrates (sugar) very quickly. This can spike your insulin level.

Imagine drinking orange juice instead of eating an orange. The digestive work is simplified, so the body does not need to use up more energy or calories to digest the food. This means that the simplified food is more fattening for you because the body does not need to work to digest it. If you were sick, this may be a good thing, so the body can spend more time healing than digesting.

For Your Wellbeing

Anatomy & Physiology of the Body's Nervous and Digestive System

The why and the how of the mind/brain function, this will inform you of why you eat the way you do.

When a baby is born, he/she will need to eat, sleep and eliminate, and they will use crying as a method of communication. Their only two natural fears are of falling and loud noises, while everything else is learned. A small child will eat what is set in front of them, or put into their grasp or mouth.

Let's explore how the body, brain and mind are connected.
As you read more details about the brain, the most important thing to remember is that it needs sugar to function! The rest of your body needs other nutrients to function properly. Guess which one will usually win?

SIMPLY PUT:

Your brain will cause you to crave certain foods, and until you acknowledge in your mind that you have a problem and need to change, this will continue.

Your brain remembers both pleasure and pain, and will do anything to stay out of the latter. Most people remember by association. The information in our memory is somehow associated with something, be it smell, taste, sight, sounds or how something feels.

Imagine an orange... fruit, color, texture, shape, smell, taste, and nutrients. Imagine as if you have it in your hands, and you placed it on a cutting board. Taking a knife you safely cut it into pieces. The dripping juice and fresh aroma are now quite noticeable. You take a piece and bite into it; the taste is sweet and succulent.

I would bet right now that your mouth has started to produce saliva in anticipation of the orange, but remember, the orange is imaginary and is only in your memory.

Do you now realize how amazing your brain is? There is no orange but your mind made your body believe there was one coming and reacted as if there was. The brain will always win!

Ask yourself these questions: "Do I have control of my memories?",

"Is my mind more powerful than my brain?", "Does my body have any control at all?".

NOW, FOR THOSE OF YOU WHO NEED MORE FACTS, HERE IS SOME MORE INFORMATION.

Those of you who get bored with the science can skim through, but there is some really good information in this section you may realize you like.

To really understand why you eat what you do, and to truly be able to change your eating habits, I would like you to understand the importance of the Nervous System. For this, you should have at least a basic understanding of how your body functions.

The Nervous System is composed of two major parts:
1st – Central Nervous System (CNS) – brain and spinal column (where memories are stored)
2nd – Peripheral Nervous System (PNS) – sensory nerves (touch) and motor nerves (movement)

QUICK OVERVIEW:

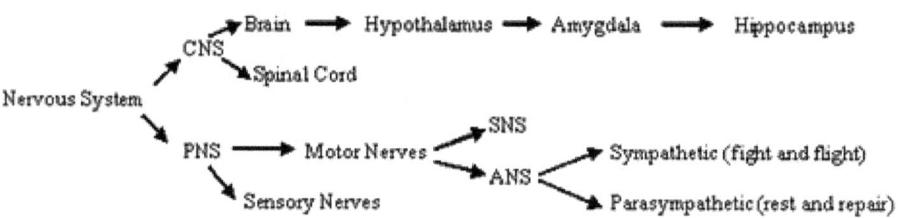

I would like you to take notice of the pathway from the CNS to hippocampus, and also the pathway from the PNS to the ANS, sympathetic and parasympathetic.
Why are they important?
The top one, CNS, is how you retain and recall your memories, and the bottom one, PNS, is how you respond to outside influences (fight or flight or rest and repair).

THE CENTRAL NERVOUS SYSTEM (CNS)

Consists of the brain and Spinal column, and is considered the supervisor of the body's nervous activity.

For example, if you are hungry to the point your stomach is growling, and you don't have anything healthy immediately available, your PNS will cause you to spot and grab whatever will get sugar to the brain the quickest, such as chips, sweets, or anything of that nature.

Scientifically speaking, the brain will send an impulse from the CNS to the PNS, and the PNS sends an impulse to the rest of the body telling it to get food.

The memory's imprint of how many times you've previously done this will play a big part in what you grab to eat. The body has a natural hibernation response, and will store fat for energy if you have starved it before.

The brain will do anything to protect itself, and starvation is a key factor. The body can't predict when you're going to feed it next, it just knows that it's hungry right now.

A diagram, for those of you who would like to see the brain and the three main parts:

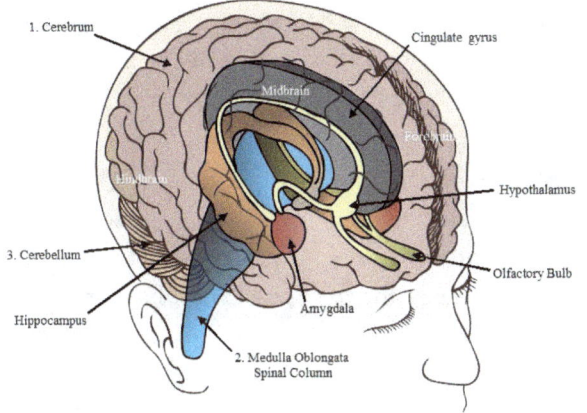

- Cerebrum (your conscious thought)
- Medulla oblongata (controls the unconscious functions of your body)
- Cerebellum (balance in your body, also unconsciously)

- The cerebrum is the largest area of the brain. (Take note of the arrow pointing to the area on top, and notice the same texture all over). The cerebrum makes up the conscious brain, and is divided into two hemispheres; the left (the analytical part of you), and the right (the creative part of you).
    - Function: our intelligence and reasoning, personality, interpretation of sensory impulses, motor function, planning and

organization, memory and touch sensation.

- The medulla oblongata is the part of the brain that connects to the spinal cord.
  - Function: Medulla oblongata regulates the unconscious functions of your body. Ie: heart rate, breathing, blood pressure, vomiting, coughing, sneezing, swallowing, and hiccupping.

- The cerebellum is the second largest part of the brain, after the cerebrum. Located at the lower back portion of your skull.
  - Function: The cerebellum coordinates balance, muscle coordination, and maintains normal muscle tone and posture.

The Peripheral Nervous System – (PNS)
Is made up of sensory and motor nerves. These nerves extend from the brain and spinal cord, linking to all other parts of the body.

Somatic Nervous System – (SNS)
The somatic nervous system is responsible for voluntary control, consciously making your body do something. Maybe you want to go get a glass of water. This is the part of the nervous system that helps tell the muscles to move, and reacts when you touch something too hot or cold.

Autonomic Nervous System – (ANS)
Normally operates without voluntary control (it is unconscious or we are unaware). Example: when you put food into your mouth and start to chew, your tongue and salivary glands are under subconscious control and receive orders from the brain via the nerves of the PNS. While you are eating you are not thinking what your pancreas, liver, or spleen are doing. Those organs are working unconsciously in your body because the medulla oblongata subconsciously instructs them.

There are two major divisions in the ANS:
- Sympathetic nerves – create fight or flight response
- Parasympathetic nerves – create rest and repair response

These two, Sympathetic and Parasympathetic, are very important to know about. Depending on how you handle outside influences, both consciously or subconsciously, will determine how your body will respond and

what foods you will choose to eat.
You have two choices in any situation, responding accordingly to your outside influences:

Sympathetic (fight and flight)

or

Parasympathetic (rest and repair)

Imagine an all you can eat dinner buffet (smells and sight of food). You have two choices, run away or relax and enjoy.

Your memory plays a big part on your decision. Your subconscious will most likely take over. If you have great memories of buffets from the past, you will likely stay and enjoy the food.

Whether or not you're hungry will also affect your decision to either stay or leave.

If you are trying to lose weight, and your memory of eating at a buffet is good, then it will take a lot of conscious concentration to walk on by or eat only healthy foods.

Can you guess which one will always win, your brain or your body? The answer is the brain!!!

Any anatomy book that deals with death of the cells and organs says the brain is the last body part to die, and it is also the most protected – think about how thick the skull is, or how protected the spinal column is. Think about when someone is sick in the hospital, and maybe unconscious. They will have an intravenous drip (usually a saline and glucose (sugar) mixture) in their arm feeding them sugar for the brain, and saline for electrolytes, to keep the body alive. Even though the person may lose a great amount of body weight, the brain does not care as long as it gets what it needs.
It is not the body that will win! It will be the brain.

Your brain is constantly adjusting and calibrating with all the experiences you are having each day, and will decide how to react… and depending on the magnitude of the experience (good, bad or blah) will determine what you eat. Past experiences may influence the decision quite a bit. Your mind and body have a memory of your past experiences, and will take the simplest solution to fix the problem.

Meaning:

If you are having any stress in your body, there will be more acid than alkaline, and with more acid, it is telling the mind and universe that the body is dying. (Acid creates death in the body and pathogens come to decompose it). If the brain goes into a sympathetic state (fight or flight response) because it thinks it is dying, the brain will crave sugar to keep it functioning. Meaning, your hand just grabbed sugar of some sort (simple carbohydrates – bread, chips, cake, cookies or chocolate) to balance the sensation of death.

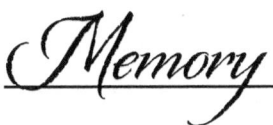

Memory

Your memories, experiences and choices are the reason that you are probably reading this book. Remember, these are just memories and are not set in stone for the rest of your life. You can change your mind and decide to eat something different anytime you choose to. To change a negative issue in your life into a positive one, you must take control! You need something, which I call a carrot, which is a more powerful reason to change to the new desired outcome.

The emotional charge associated with any negative past experience can hold you back from choosing a new eating habit (unless you have any physical issue due to drugs, alcohol, surgery or hormones), but that emotional charge can be changed. If you have a chemical imbalance, or had surgery, you will most likely be able to change your pattern; it might take a bit longer and more effort though.

For those of you who love knowledge and details, here is more information on how and where these memories are stored. For those of you that have had enough information already, just skim through and read the paragraphs that interest you the most.

MEMORY

The brain has the ability to store, retain, and subsequently retrieve information through our daily senses of touch, sight, smell, taste and sound.

Memories are stored in the limbic system, which is in the cerebrum. The main parts that control this action are the hypothalamus, amygdala, hippocampus and thalamus.

The good or bad experiences that you sense during the day are noticed by the hypothalamus, and are stored for the day in the amygdala. At night when you sleep this stored information is scanned and sorted in the hippocampus (some say that is how your dreams are formed). The most important memories are stored for future retrieval, and the remainder of the day's information is erased.

Limbic System

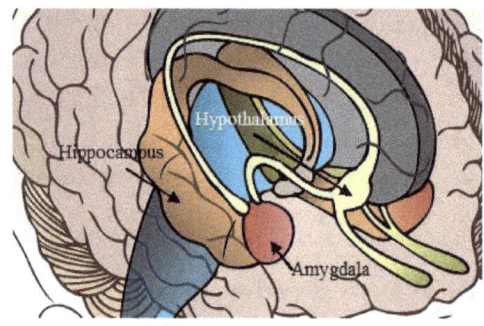

There are three structures: the hypothalamus, amygdala, and the hippocampus, which are in the middle part of the brain.

Hypothalamus

The hypothalamus controls our motivated behaviours, like thermal regulation, sexuality, combativeness, hunger and thirst. The hypothalamus plays a major role in our emotions, specifically pleasure, rage, aversion, displeasure and the tendency for loud, uncontrollable laughter.

However, the hypothalamus has more to do with the expression (symptomatic – fight or flight) of emotions.

When you have an emotional feeling (such as laughing, crying, or fear) the brain will scan the limbic system for any past memory that has a similar experience and, once found, will trigger the body to react 'fight or flight' or 'rest and repair'. Depending on your past memories, your body will react by leaving the scene or staying to enjoy the experience. Have you ever been at a meal and did not want to eat everything on your plate, but because your upbringing taught you it was impolite not to you ate everything anyways? You reacted on your feelings and memories, not by your own conscious control.

Amygdala

The amygdala resembles a little almond, deep inside the brain, which connects with the hippocampus and the thalamus.

These connections make it possible for the amygdala to play its important role on the mediation and expression of your emotions, such as friendship, love, affection, fear, rage and aggression. It can also identify danger.

People with marked lesions or scarring of the amygdala have lost memory. One example would be the recognition of a well known person to them. They really do know exactly who the other person is, but are not capable of deciding (or remembering) whether he likes or dislikes the person.

HIPPOCAMPUS

The hippocampus is particularly involved with memory phenomena, especially the formation of long-term memory (memories that can last forever).

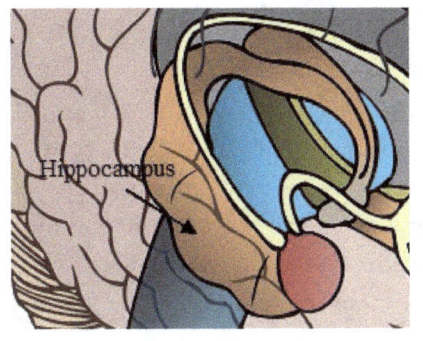

When both hippocampi (right and left) are destroyed, nothing can be retained in the memory. The person quickly forgets any recently received message. An intact hippocampus allows a person to compare a present situation with a similar past experience(s), therefore being able to choose the best option.

Thinking about why you need to know this in so much detail? Not all of you will care to really understand this information, but those of you who truly desire to change your eating habits will need to understand how you ended up at this moment in time, and what is compelling you to stay this way.

There are three types of memories that you should know about: long term, short term and working memory. The first two types of memories control who you are, and if you are in conscious control of your eating habits!

LONG-TERM MEMORY can disappear by what is considered the natural forgetting process. To retain a memory for a long, long time, the thought or experience you want to remember would need to have made a major impact on you (good or bad), or you would have to do something repetitively so it becomes habit.

Did you know that long-term memory can last as little as a few days, or as long as decades?

SHORT-TERM MEMORY is said to hold a small amount of information for about 20-30 seconds. The information held in short-term memory may be recently processed information, or information recently retrieved from long-term memory.

WORKING MEMORY is when you are consciously working on a project and are reading, writing or talking about information that you may decide later to keep as short or long term memory. An example is an exam. You need the answers for the test, but not necessarily will you keep the answers for long thereafter.

NOW FOR SOME REALLY INTERESTING INFORMATION ON HOW YOUR MEMORIES ARE STORED

Scientists say that we only consciously retain about 9 bits of information (outside stimulus) every second, and even that is still a lot of information for the brain to deal with. As talked about before, this daily information is stored in the amygdala during the waking hours, and at night when you sleep this information gets sorted. Information that the mind decides to keep goes to the hippocampus for long term memory, and the information not needed is erased.

Your brain mostly remembers pleasure and pain.

Think of an orange... color, size, texture; cutting it open and noticing the juices, the smell, and the thought of its sweet taste. Did your mouth start salivating again?

The brain will always win!

Most of us have control of our limbic system, but we don't have enough practice in using it efficiently.

There are two things you must be aware of for you to be in control of your memory.

- 1st — SAME STATE OF AWARENESS is where the body and mind are feeling the same awareness of the surroundings as it was at another time.

Imagine it is Christmas or Thanksgiving, and you are at a family gathering having dinner. The familiar smells of turkey, stuffing and all the other trimmings fill the air.

Now notice if you are salivating again triggering the body to react as if the food is right there in front of you. Now your body is getting ready to eat this imaginary food.

Your memories are a very interesting factor in your weight control.

Some of you do not even consciously eat; some eat to get rid of feelings, while others eat to feel them.

      Pleasure or pain... are you happy or sad to be at this family gathering?

- 2nd — You need a <u>PLAN</u> of the food you are going to eat no matter what state you are in. Be it breakfast, lunch, snack, dinner or supper. Write the plan out, or at least mentally prepare ahead of time what you are going to eat.

A habit takes 21 to 42 days to form, or break, and sometimes it needs to be repeated months later (depending on how long the habit has been practiced in the past). Most addicts already know this. It doesn't take much to break the good intentions of quitting something, be it drugs, alcohol, a relationship or food.

What it comes down to is...
Most of us love to feel good... pleasure and pain
And the brain will always win.

You will only change your eating habits when:
- You admit that you have a problem, and realize that there is a better way
- The bad eating habit becomes destructive, and the doctor tells you to change

Each and every day, you have to choose to be aware of your eating habits and decide to change the feelings that are controlling you. Realise that you do have the power to change your mind. Your mind is considered a very different part from your brain.

The Mind

The Mind is considered to be inside the brain

Definition:
The element of a person that enables them to be aware of the world and their experiences, to think and to feel; the faculty of consciousness and thought.

There are three factors that make up the mind: conscious, subconscious and superconscious.

Conscious Mind
(most of us think we are in control of our lives)
- The state of being aware of and responsive to one's surroundings
- Acts as a filter for thought or outside influences
- Stored in the amygdala (limbic system)
- Thinks or analyzes information
- Controls our movements
- Organizes responsibilities
- Processes 7 trillion to 9 trillion (9,000,000,000.00) bits of information every second. We consciously only notice about 9 bits.
- In seconds (response time):
    - From sight to touch – 0.071
    - From touch to sight – 0.053
    - From sight to hearing – 0.16
    - From hearing to sight – 0.06
    - From one ear to another – 0.064

Subconscious Mind
(the part of you that's really in control of your life)
- Of or concerning the part of the mind of which one is not fully aware, but which influences one's actions and feelings.
- Stored in the hippocampus (limbic system)

- Stores your belief system, self image, morals, habits, emotions, fears, secrets and memories
- Cannot tell the difference between real or imagined
- Understands subliminal messages
- Ability to solve problems creatively
- Dreams
- Some believe your psychic ability is accessed here

SUPERCONSCIOUS MIND
(the part of you that God sends messages to)
- Transcending human or normal consciousness (Higher power)
- Higher self
- Accessible through meditation, yoga, breathing and hypnosis
- Group consciousness or God consciousness
- Healing
- All knowing, higher power
- Akasha records (spiritual knowledge of past, present and future events) can be obtained
- Brilliant ideas, music, art, movies, stories, concepts are formatted here – Einstein, Nostradamus, etc

The mind is what makes us who we are, and our beliefs or judgments of pleasure and pain dictate our next move.

Now that you have admitted that you have an eating problem, (you have admitted that to yourself, right?) and eating this way is not doing you any good, then let's move on to the digestive system

Anatomy/Physiology of the Digestive System and Nutrition

Nutritional Role of the Digestive System
The functions of the digestive system are to:

- Process food, supplying nutrients to fuel the body's organs and systems.
- To eliminate wastes from the body.

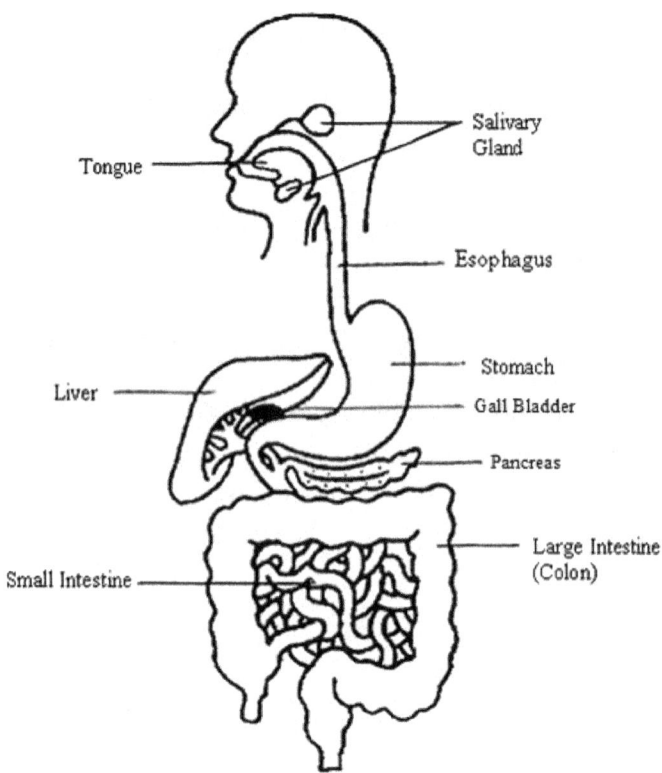

Simply Put
- From your mouth to rectum takes anywhere from twenty-four to thirty-six hours.
- You put food into your mouth

- Your teeth chew the food and break it down into smaller pieces. The better you chew your food the faster it can be digested, and more nutrients will be absorbed.
- The saliva in your mouth has enzymes, which help to break down the food
- The food goes into the stomach, which takes minutes to many hours to churn. More juices and enzymes are released to help break the food down into a liquid substance.
- Next, the food goes into the duodenum, and digestive liquids are secreted from the pancreas and gallbladder to break down the food even further.
- IMPORTANT INFORMATION! The food particles need to be as small as liquid particles for the body to absorb the nutrients.
- The brain takes about 20 minutes to register that the stomach is full.
- The small intestine, which is approximately twenty two feet long will absorb the liquid sized nutrients for the rest of the body.
- Then, onto the large intestine, or colon (three feet in length), to re-absorb any water from the food fibers. At this point, the fibers are getting ready to be eliminated from your body.
- The ileocecal valve, located between the small and large intestine, stops the food particles from going back up and being absorbed in the small intestine.
- And then out through your rectum, and flushed away forever.

An interesting fact about eating

Any time you put something into your mouth, the brain will think it is food and get ready to eat.

Imagine you just ate a very delicious and nutritious evening meal.

I need you to remember that it takes about twenty minutes for the food to start to go through the stomach and reach the small intestine. The food that is in the small intestine is really important because all the nutrients are being transferred to the rest of the body from this area.

You wait a while for dessert, maybe half an hour or more. Now what did you just do? You just told the body to get ready because new food is coming and so what does it do? It starts to flush the really healthy food you just ate quickly through the stomach and small intestine to get ready for the new food coming. All those great nutrients are now being quickly moved and being replaced by the dessert nutrients, which you will probably go to bed with.

You would have been better off eating the dessert first, as long as you left room for the nutritious food to go to bed with. That way the good nutrients are left for the body to digest at bedtime.

The next big tease for the digestive system is gum and candy. These types of candies trick the body into believing that food is coming, when nothing actually does. The juices and enzymes your body produces can cause issues because no food really came, but all the enzymes did. Also, you had better not swallow your gum, because it can clog up the villi, which absorb the nutrients in the small intestine!!!

FOR THOSE OF YOU WHO NEED MORE FACTS, HERE IS A WHOLE LOT MORE.

Again those of you who do not require this information just skip on by.
- The digestive system is made up of a mucous membrane similar to the type located in the respiratory and genitourinary systems. The digestive system resembles a disassembly line that works to extract vital parts from whole nutritional materials. Food is broken down by digestive juices into small, easily absorbed nutrients. It generates the energy required to maintain a healthy body.
- For a healthy and efficient body to be maintained, the food content needs to be both balanced and nutritious. We are responsible for our own basic health. The old adage "we are what we eat" is true in many cases. Because of this, we need to understand some of the ways in which it can go wrong.

The body requires raw material to grow and repair itself, as well as for heat and energy. These raw materials are supplied in the form of food that comes in a variety of packages we ingest and convert into compounds, which generate and sustain life.

Digestive Process

The entire digestive process is controlled from start to the finish by the hypothalamus (what an amazing part of the brain). This includes the sensation of hunger, and the emptying of the bowels.

Digestion involves the breaking down of organic compounds into simple soluble substances absorbable by the tissues. The process involves catalytic reactions between ingested food and enzymes secreted into the intestinal tract. Digestion of fatty substances appears to require the involvement of bile salts, phospholipids, fatty acids and monoglycerides. Other nutrients, such as iron and vitamin B 12, are absorbable by specific "carrier proteins" that make them transferable by intestinal cells.

Digestion includes both mechanical and chemical functions. The mechanical functions include chewing, the churning action of the stomach and intestinal peristaltic action. These forces move the food through the digestive tract and mix it with various secretions.

Three chemical reactions occur: conversion of carbohydrates into simple sugars, the breakdown of protein into amino acids, and conversion of fats into fatty acids and glycerol.

The six salivary glands produce secretions that mix with the food. The saliva breaks down starches into dextrin and maltose, dissolves solid food to make it susceptible to the action of later intestinal secretions, stimulates secretion of digestive enzymes and lubricates the mouth and esophagus.

RATE OF DIGESTION

It takes between twenty minutes to six hours for a meal to be converted from solids to semi-liquids in the stomach. The rate at which the stomach moves food is controlled primarily by the duodenum. The sphincter releases hormones that control the muscle movements of the stomach, and so regulates the rate of digestion. As a result, the duodenum receives the chyme gradually, in just the right amount, for optimum digestion and absorption. When the stomach is full, it signals for the release of the peptide hormone gastrin, which speeds up digestion.

Digestive Tract

The average adult has a digestive tract that is about thirty feet long from one end to the other, and can be described as a strong and continuous muscular tube. It consists of and starts at:

1. the mouth (and passes through)
2. the larynx
3. the esophagus
4. the stomach
5. the small intestine
6. the large intestine
7. (and ends at) the rectum

Taste

Although the taste buds combine to make a myriad of different flavours, there are believed to be only four primary tastes: bitter, sour, salty and sweet.

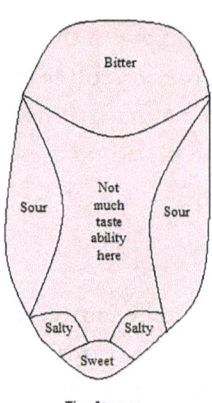

Tip of tongue

Various parts of the tongue have taste buds that are especially sensitive to one of the basic sensations of taste. You taste salt and mainly sweet on the front of the tongue, sour on the sides and bitter at the back, while the middle of the tongue registers almost no taste.

Taste is highly relative, and different people will be attracted to different foods and flavours. Aspects of taste can be hereditary, as some genes make the receptors for bitterness especially keen. In these people, saccharin is likely to produce a strong sensation of bitterness.

Each person's saliva has its own special taste, which in turn affects the taste of food. If, for example, your saliva has a low sodium content, food containing a given amount of salt would taste saltier to you than to someone whose saliva is high in sodium.

The tongue is needed in the chewing process of your food, turning and moving it to each side for the teeth to grind and break down, and moving the food to the back of the mouth to be swallowed.

Interesting fact, the more you chew real foods the better and sweeter the taste will become, and the more you chew processed foods they become bland or bitter. Try it if you don't believe me. Meat, veggies and fruit will become sweeter as you chew, but cookies, cakes, candies and most processed foods will become bland or bitter.

To enhance taste, every so often take ¼ to ½ teaspoon of sesame seed oil and swirl it on your tongue for a minute or two (you can spit it out after or swallow it).

Salivary Glands

There are three pairs of salivary glands:
1. The parotid glands, found in front of and a little below the ears. You may have become familiar with this gland when you were a child. These glands swell when you have the mumps. Swollen or not, these are the largest salivary glands.
2. The sublingual glands, situated just below the tongue, are smaller than the Parotid glands, about the size of a walnut.
3. The submandibular glands, situated below the mandible, they are the smallest of the salivary glands.

The salivary glands produce secretions containing the starch-reducing enzymes, ptyalin, which help in the digestion of cooked starches. The conversion is accomplished by a digestive enzyme known as salivary amylase, or ptyalin. Of course, saliva does a lot more than just break down starches into sugars. Without saliva, you would find it very difficult to swallow. The mucous in saliva adheres to the food and moistens it during chewing. This enables it to slide easily down the esophagus. Another function of the saliva is to keep the mouth healthy, because it is also a mild germicide. Saliva kills bacteria, especially the kind that causes tooth decay.

Peristalsis

The movement of food along the digestive tract is made possible by the wave-like motion made by the smooth muscles of the digestive system, and is known as peristalsis. The action is from the outside of the digestive tubes inwards and downwards, so that the food is forced further along the tube.

STOMACH

The stomach is a curved muscular sac-like structure that is an enlargement of the alimentary canal between the esophagus and the small intestine. It adds acids and mixes them together with the foods. Its size and shape varies with its contents and muscular tone. If it is empty, its shape is like a "J" with practically no cavity at all as the sides press inward. When full, it takes the shape of a boxing glove and the average adult stomach can hold up to 1.5 liters of food. The stomach has the ability to absorb water, certain salts, alcohol and some drugs and crystalloids.

The stomach presents two curvatures, the greater and lesser curvature. For the purpose of description it is divided into three parts:
- The cardiac portion
- The body
- The pyloric

The openings into the stomach are guarded by circular bands of muscle, like purse strings, with the cardiac sphincter muscles at the entrance and the pylorus sphincter muscle at the exit. The cardiac sphincter prevents acid and ingested food from backing up, and the pylorus sphincter muscle prevents food from leaving the stomach prematurely. Each ball of food, or bolus, enters the part of the stomach called the fundus and pushes food previously eaten down and out towards the stomach walls. The fundus and the main body of the stomach serve as a storage area, holding food until it is time for it to move along to the antrum and the duodenum (pronounced "du-o-dee-num").

The stomach has four coats or coverings:
1. An outer coat of serous membrane.
2. A middle muscular coat made up of longitudinal, circular and oblique muscle fibers.
3. A submucous coat.
4. A mucous coat or membrane which forms the inner lining.

The mucous membrane is arranged in folds or rugae, which disappear when the stomach is distended. The membrane is lined with glands, which produce gastric juice. This contains hydrochloric acid and some enzymes, including pepsin, rennin and lipase. Pepsin breaks proteins into peptones and proteoses. Rennin separates milk into liquid and solid portions. The lipase acts on fat.

The middle muscular coat contains a network of blood vessels that nourish the structure, as well as nerves that activate glands and muscles. The muscles move, soften and mix the food with the secretions and push it out into the small intestine when it is a thick, soupy consistency.

The hydrochloric acid the stomach secretes is corrosive enough to dissolve a razor blade or annihilate living cells. Sometimes it actually eats into the stomach itself and creates ulcers. Usually, however, the stomach remains impervious to attack. The gastric lining is coated with mucous, which forms a barrier between the acid and the stomach walls. The mucous is somewhat alkaline, and neutralizes the acid to keep the stomach from digesting itself. Furthermore, the stomach lining sheds cells at the rate of half a million cells per minute, and replaces them so rapidly that the stomach essentially has a new lining every three days. Even if hydrochloric acid does damage the cells, the stomach makes repairs automatically.

The presence of food in the stomach stimulates the production of gastric secretions. Some constituents of secretions only act when exposed to the alkalinity of the small intestine. The stomach has a pyloric valve at the point where it merges with the small intestine which controls the releases of the partially digested food material. Watery foods, such as soup, leave the stomach quite quickly, while fats remain considerably longer. An ordinary mixed meal is emptied from the stomach between 20 minutes and 4 hours. Foods rich in carbohydrates leave the stomach faster than proteins, and proteins more rapidly than fats.

The stomach gradually releases materials into the upper small intestine, where digestion is completed.

Small Intestine

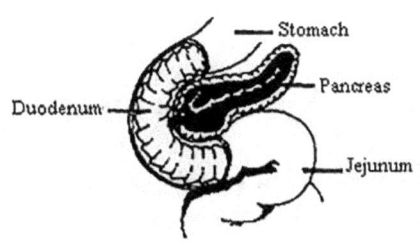

The main food processing and assimilation of proteins takes place in the small intestine.

From the stomach, the food passes into the duodenum, which is about ten inches long and shaped like the letter "C". As food enters the duodenum from the stomach, it stimulates the following three organs to release the chemicals needed to finish digestion:

- The gallbladder stores and releases bile.

- The pancreas produces an alkaline juice to neutralize acid.
- The liver performs many actions and will be described in more detail later in this section.

These three organs (liver, pancreas and gallbladder) fluids neutralize the gastric acid, ending the gastric phase of digestion.

The small intestine pours forth mucous to protect the duodenum from damage by gastric acid. It also produces hormones that stimulate the liver, pancreas and gallbladder to release digestive substances.

The remainder of the small intestine comprises the "jejunum", pronounced "je- joo-num", which is about eight feet long, and the ileum, which is about twelve feet long. The inner coat of the small intestine is comprised of mucous membrane, arranged in folds known as valvulae conniventes, and unlike the rugae of the stomach these folds do not disappear with the distension of the intestines. The convoluted surface of the intestine amounts to 140 sq. m. or 1500 sq. feet in an adult. The total length of the small intestine is 6.7 to 7.6 meters, or 22 to 25 feet.

The mucous membrane is covered with minute finger-like projections known as villi. Each villi contains a lacteal for the absorption of fat, and a capillary for the absorption of sugar and protein.

This mucous membrane also contains intestinal glands, which produce a secretion known as succus entericus. This secretion contains enzymes for the digestion of proteins and sugars. The mucous membrane is studded with lymphatic nodes, and it is in the latter part of the small intestine, known as the ileum, that groups of these nodules are found. These are called peyer's patches. The function of the peyer's patches is to fight infection.

The small intestine then merges with the large intestine. Although wider than the small intestine, the large intestine is much shorter, a total of 1.5 - 1.8 metres (meters), or 5 - 6 feet long.

LARGE INTESTINE (COLON)

The majority of nutrient absorption takes place in the small intestine, while the large intestine re-circulates the water.

The colon, or large intestine, has the ability to absorb water, certain salts, alcohol and some drugs and crystalloids. Certain whole proteins are also believed to pass through the intestinal barrier.

For the purpose of this description, the large intestine is divided into the following nine parts:
1. Caecum (Cecum), with the ileocecal valve (the valve prevents backflow).

2. Ascending colon (passes up the right side of the abdomen).
3. Hepatic flexure (bends sharply to the left in the area of the liver).
4. Transverse colon (crosses the abdomen: right to left just under the ribs).
5. Splenic flexure (bends sharply downward in the area of the spleen).
6. Descending colon (passes down the left side of the abdomen).
7. Sigmoid flexure (bends sharply to the right and backwards).
8. Sigmoid colon (moves down and back to the rectum).
9. Rectum and anus (the rectum is 25 - 50 mm, or 5 - 6 inches long, and is the exit, of which is guarded by two sphincter muscles known as the anus).

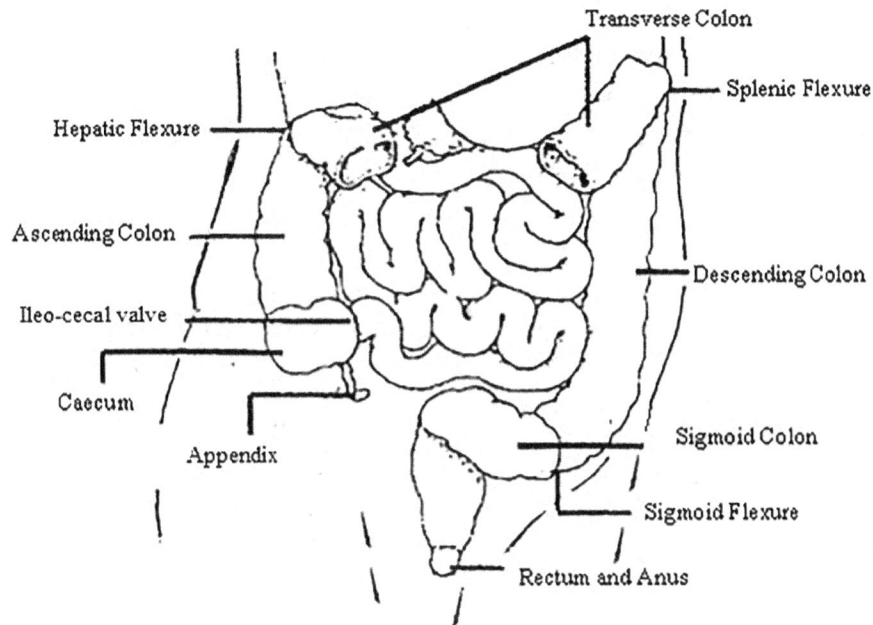

NOTE: Although the diagram indicates the appendix, it is not technically part of the large intestine. It is simply an organ attached to the large intestine with its own role to play, separate from that of the large intestine.

Does death begin in the colon?

Many years ago I was in a practitioner's waiting room, and I started to read an article that asked this question. Does death begin in the colon? There was a test to take to find out how healthy your large intestine was.

Here is that test, a self analysis of your intestinal health.

Directions:
- Check only one answer for each question.
- After each answer you check, you will find a number in brackets. Transfer this number to the line provided.
- Add up all the numbers you transferred to the score column to get your total score.

Questions
1. How many hours does it usually take your food to digest (move from mouth to elimination)? If you eat corn on the cob you will know how long it takes.
    - a. Less than 24 hours (0)
    - b. 24-36 hours (1)
    - c. More than 36 hours (0)   _____

2. How many bowel movements did you have yesterday?
    - a. None (0)
    - b. One or two (1)
    - c. Three (2)   _____

3. How long are your stools usually?
    - a. The size of pellets or small granulated flakes (0)
    - b. Shorter than a foot (0)
    - c. About a foot long (1)   _____

4. How large are your stools around?
	a. Less than a silver dollar or toonie (0)
	b. About the size of a silver dollar or toonie (1)
	c. Larger than a silver dollar or toonie (0) _____

5. What colour are your stools usually?
	a. Light brown (1)
	b. Green, red, black or any colour other than light brown (0) _____

6. How much undigested food can you see in your stools?
	a. A lot (0)
	b. A little (1)
	c. None at all (2) _____

7. Do your bowel movements usually float or sink or both?
	a. Float - Horizontally (0)
	b. Sink (0)
	c. Both float and sink at the same time (1). _____

8. How often do you have cold hands and feet?
	a. Very often (0)
	b. Occasionally (1)
	c. Never (2) _____

9. Can you see mucous in your stools or coating them?
	a. Often (0)
	b. Occasionally (1)
	c. Never (2) _____

Add up and put your total score here

_____

- A higher score indicates greater intestinal health; a score of 12 is highest, 0 is lowest.
- A lower score indicates that you may want to consider the services of a professional colon cleansing practitioner, discuss these questions with your doctor, or possibly have a baseline colonoscopy.

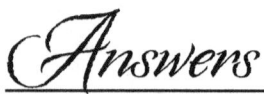

Answers

1. Food should move through you at a relatively even rate of speed. Digestion begins with peristaltic action initiated by chewing and continues until elimination. In a healthy colon, this takes 24-36 hours. If your food goes through faster, it usually indicates an accumulated layer of debris preventing your colon from digesting food. If digestion takes more time, then impactions or distortions are usually slowing the process.

2. You should have one bowel movement roughly 24-36 hours after every meal, or three a day if you eat three meals per day.

3. The length of your stools should conform to the segment lengths of a clean and healthy colon. Each segment, ascending, transverse and descending are about one foot long. Passed stool tends to break at the segment junctures. A healthy stool is thus about a foot long. A shorter stool usually indicates the colon is unable to process food properly where the stool does not have the right moisture balance.

4. The diameter of the colon should be roughly that of a silver dollar. Smaller indicates constriction, perhaps due to prolonged stress or accumulated layers of uneliminated debris. Larger indicates lack of colon muscle tone from lack of exercise, low assimilation of minerals or a low fiber diet.

5. Your stool should be composed of 95-98% dead bacteria and 2-5% fiber that has not broken down. Dead bacteria are light brown and the healthy stool is thusly light brown. Other colours can indicate the presence of undigested food or, in some cases, blood. Stool can also be off-colour as a result of taking medication or vitamins.

6. A healthy colon produces stool with no sign of undigested food. Undigested food particles usually means accumulated debris is preventing proper digestion.

7. Healthy stool half floats and half sinks in water. Stool that floats entirely is usually filled with undigested fat or gas. Stool that sinks usually has undigested minerals, or is so compact from retention it contains little moisture.

8. The composting function of the colon is a major source of body heat. The internal temperature of a healthy colon is roughly 105 degrees Fahrenheit or 41 degrees Celsius, allowing the colon to serve as the body's radiant heater. While there are a number of reasons why your hands and feet might be cold, most common is chronic constipation, indicating the colon is not processing food fast enough to produce heat.

9. Mucous in or coating your stool can mean a number of things: possibly a colitis condition, infection or irritation. A person in a detoxification cycle after a fasting regime will also find mucous in or coating stool eliminated from a healthy colon. Under most conditions, however, you cannot observe mucous in or coating stools eliminated from a healthy colon.

THIS ARTICLE IS PRESENTED AS A PUBLIC SERVICE. AFTER READING, PLEASE PASS IT TO A FRIEND. YOU MAY SAVE A LIFE.
FOR MORE INFORMATION OR A COLONIC SESSION, LOOK IN YOUR HEALTH FOOD STORE INFO, NATURAL MAGAZINES, NATURAL OR ALTERNATIVE HEALTH IN YOUR YELLOW PAGES.

I took this test back in 1987, and my total was barely a five. I took a copy of the test home and my husband ended up being an eleven. I couldn't believe it, I thought he lied. I went back to the natural health clinic and had a colonic, since the test revealed how bad my digestion was.

A colonic is not as bad as you may think. You remove your pants and underwear, and lay on your side on a table with a towel draped over you. When the practitioner comes in he/she applies a bit of petroleum jelly to your anus and inserts a small metal apparatus that has two tubes. One that is connected to body temperature filtered water, and the other to remove the wash.

The practitioner allows some water to flow into the rectum through the tube and counts, and then removes the water. They will repeat this many times.

> ONE SECRET TO THE SESSION IS TO LET GO AND RELAX. IF YOU START TO HOLD ON AND WILL NOT ALLOW YOUR BODY TO ELIMINATE AND YOU ARE WASTING YOUR SESSION.

To my astonishment, my practitioner told me exactly what I had eaten the night before. She was looking at the clear tube while the debris moved through (part of their job). I was informed that I did not chew my food enough, as there was still solid food coming through. This meant the nutrients were not being absorbed into my body and the large debris was not healthy for my system. She also told me that they can tell if a person has parasites (which, thank God, I did not).

Half way through the hour long session you are asked to turn onto your back with knees bent and feet flat. The practitioner rubs your stomach in a clockwise motion to help manually move any debris in the large intestine to be eliminated.

Once the session is completed you get off the table and sit on the toilet to eliminate any excess of water, lifting your arms above your head and turning your torso slowly from side to side to help release any excess.

I was told it may take anywhere from one to eight sessions to cleanse the large intestine, and a person will feel much more energetic afterwards. I ended up needing three (I knew because after the third session I was a twelve out of twelve on the test).

A year later I did three more sessions because I hadn't changed my eating habits and my bowel was clogged again. After that, I changed a lot of what I ate and chewed my food better. The next time I went it was three years later, and only needed one session; then again five years after for one more.

You will be told to take an acidophilus supplement to offset the natural bacteria that was removed from the session. You need these good bacteria to kill and break down the particles in the large intestine.

A few years later, I started working at the clinic and was amazed at how many cancer clients came in to receive colonics, cleansing their body so that it didn't have to work so hard at digestion and could focus on the body's immune system.

The difference between a professional colonic with three to eight sessions and an enema is the colonic will be able to cleanse your whole large intestine, where as an enema will only do about six inches.

Not only can you have the benefit of a clean colon and more energy, a colonic will clean out any toxic waste. Your eyesight, skin, muscles, joints, heart, headaches, emotions, memory, sleep, and genitor-urinary system may all be improved.

As quoted: "In short, when the intestines are clean and functioning normally, we are healthy and happy. But let them stagnate and they will distil the poisons of decay, poisoning every organ of the body. As a result we age prematurely."

From this evidence we can say that death truly can begin in the colon.

Psychology of the Colon

Reprinted from an article by John Harvey Kellogg, M.D.

"The colon is richly supplied with nerves and is highly sensitive to influence by all emotions, pleasurable or the opposite. Studies have shown that unpleasant emotions of all sorts can stop peristalsis (wave like motion of the muscles in the digestive tract). Even very slight emotional excitement, as slight as anxiety, annoyance, apprehension, or ill-temper may stop all movement of the intestines, as well as of the stomach together with gastric secretions.

The colon, like the face, responds to every passing emotion. The intestines are perhaps more sensitive than are the muscles of the face to emotional excitement because they are more richly supplied with blood vessels and sympathetic nerves.

X-ray studies of animals have demonstrated the intimate association of the colon with the sympathetic nervous system, and the profound effect of all forms of emotional excitement. When a dog was placed in a strange surrounding, peristalsis within its colon ceased for several hours. When a cat, while under observation, had its tail pinched, peristalsis also ceased. The movements did not begin again until the cat was pacified and purring contentedly.

The depressing influence of fear is well established. The frightened colon cannot discharge its contents because the descending colon is in a spastic state. So long as the person is fearful that his bowels will not move, they will not. The colon is in a state of fright. It is crippled, but all that is needed for a cure may be to get rid of apprehension and fear. In such a case, the most effective remedies will not move the bowels until the element of fear is removed. Confidence and faith can change the situation.
The angry colon shuts up like a clam and declares "No Thoroughfare Here". Some persons are obstinately constipated because of a chronic state of ill will or anger.

Grief shuts up the outlet of the body's sewage as tightly as does fear or anger. The worried colon neither secrets nor contracts. Both secretion and contraction are needed for efficient action-secretion for lubrication, and contraction for transportation of the food residues to the exit. Loss of sleep, business worries, domestic trial, or harassment from any cause may render the colon dysfunctional.

In view of these facts, which might be multiplied at great length, it is evident that a right mental attitude as well as roughage and lubrication are essential for the successful treatment of the sluggish colon. With the various food accessories might be mingled the firm faith that the natural and biological means employed will accomplish the desired outcome.

Such faith should lead to regular visits to the toilet at the times when the bowels should move, that is, rising in the morning and before going to bed at night. Do not wait for "the call" but invite the call by giving the colon a chance for evacuation, and by all means, avoid haste. A hurried visit to the toilet will not encourage normal colon activity. A slow colon must be given time, especially when by a change in diet and attention to colon hygiene it is just beginning to behave in something like a normal manner. By patient training, the sluggish bowel may be trained to act with natural promptness and celerity (speed).

From early infancy, the habit of prompt attention to the call for evacuation of the colon should be assiduously cultivated. Instead of doing this, the child is usually subjected to a process of housebreaking, much like that to which house dogs are subjected. The result is the derangement of the natural order that emptied the colon after each meal, or three or four times a day. This established a crippled condition of the colon that permits but one evacuation a day, a form of constipation that is so universal among civilized people that it has come to be regarded as natural.

As soon as the child begins to run about, the mother begins to train him to restrain movements of his bowel and bladder to suit convenience of time and place. A false sense of modesty also becomes a restraining influence that soon upsets the normal intestinal rhythm, laying foundation for lifelong constipation and all the miseries associated with these conditions and the autointoxication to which they give rise.

Indeed, the majority of people and many physicians regard regularity as the essential element of colon health, and almost ignore the matter of frequency and thoroughness of evacuation. The late Sir Lauser Brunton, an eminent English internist told of a lady who answered his enquiry about her colon function "Perfectly regular Sir, perfectly regular." When further questioned, she disclosed the fact that although bowel movements were perfectly regular, they occurred only once in three weeks."

Dr. Kellogg founded the Battle Creek, Michigan, Sanitarium and the Kellogg's Breakfast Cereal Company.

*** If by chance you do have parasites of any kind they are actually quite easy to get rid of. You might want to check to see if you have parasites; anyone with small children, pets or loves to garden most likely has them.

Great books to read on parasites are

"A Cure for all Diseases", by Hulda Regehr Clark
or
"Guess What Came To Dinner", by Ann Gittleman.

A couple of natural foods that rid parasites are pumpkin seeds and walnuts. There are also many parasite cleanses that you can purchase at a natural health or vitamin store.

Rectum and Anus-Excretion

The stool or undigested material is held in the rectum until excreted through the anus. Waste material or undigested food is formed into a solid mass in the colon by absorption of water into the body. If the excretory mass is propelled through the colon too quickly, it will remain semi-liquid or diarrhea. On the other hand, too slow of a movement through the colon results in constipation.

Two Other Essential Organs to the Digestive System

The liver

The liver is an organ and a gland, and is situated in the right hand side of the body just below the diaphragm. The largest organ in the body other than skin, it measures about ten to twelve inches across, and six to seven inches from the back to front, weighing approximately three and one half pounds. Protected by the rib cage, it is divided into two lobes, the large right lobe and the smaller left lobe over-laying the stomach where it joins the esophagus.

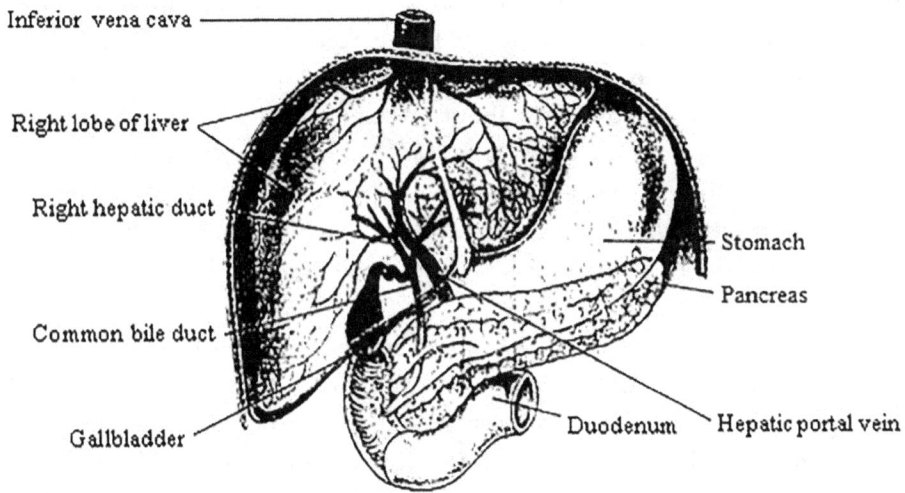

The right lobe is much larger than the left, and is subdivided into three sections. The liver can function even if as much as 90% of it was removed, and is known to re-grow. However, if the liver is destroyed by disease, the only hope for survival would be a liver transplant. Because of its many functions, it is unlikely that a machine could do all of its work. The liver is one of the few organs capable of repairing itself to be fully functional again, given time and a change in lifestyle.

The liver has many functions, one of which is the formation of bile. The liver produces up to two pints of bile each day. This passes along to the gallbladder, which is a muscular pear shaped sac about three inches long. Its function is to store bile and to concentrate it, which it does between eight to ten times. Then, when required, the bile passes out of the gallbladder into the duodenum.

Vitamins A, B, E, and K are stored in the liver. All but the B vitamins are soluble in fats and are, therefore, absorbed into the body with fatty materials. The detergent action of bile in the small intestine breaks down these fats, along with the vitamins, into suspended globules that are absorbed through the intestinal wall into the blood via lymph vessels. Without bile, the body would be deficient in its vital stockpile of vitamins. The water-soluble substances, including minerals, amino acids and carbohydrates, are transferred into the venous drainage of the intestine, and through the portal blood channels directly to the liver.

It is worth noting that a healthy liver removes a yellow pigment called bilirubin from the blood, converts it to a form that can be excreted into bile, and eliminates it from the body. A diseased liver, however, cannot do that, so the pigment remains in the bloodstream, and the skin and the whites of the eyes take on the yellowish tinge called 'jaundice'. It is interesting to note that when people talk about "yellow jaundice", they are repeating themselves, because the term 'jaundice' is derived from the word that means 'yellow'. Bilirubin is a waste product from the destruction of worn-out red blood cells. Under normal conditions, it gives the stool its characteristic colour. When a person has jaundice, the urine and tears darken, but the stool becomes lighter.

It has already been said that the liver manufactures bile, but it has a variety of other functions as well. It is a powerful detoxifying organ, breaking down many kinds of toxic molecules and rendering them harmless. It is a reservoir for blood, a storage organ for some vitamins and digested carbohydrates in the form of glycogen, which it releases to sustain blood and sugar levels. It manufactures enzymes, cholesterol, proteins, vitamin A from carotene, blood coagulation factors and other elements.

Bile is a complex fluid containing, amongst other things, bile salts and bile pigments. The pigment is derived from the disintegration of red blood cells, and it is these which give the yellow brown colour to feces when excreted, while the bile salts are reabsorbed and reused. The salts promote efficient digestion of fats by a detergent action, which gives very fine emulsification of fatty materials.

PANCREAS

The Greek name pancreas means 'all flesh' or 'all meat'. The pancreas is a cream coloured gland, 6-8 inches long and about 1 ½ inches wide. Resembling a fish with a large head and a long tail, the pancreas extends across the body, behind the stomach, in the upper left side of the abdomen. The larger end of it rests next to the duodenum. The function of the pancreas is to secrete enzymes and hormones, including insulin, needed for the digestion and absorption of food. Insulin is manufactured by cells known as the islets of Langerhans, which are scattered like little islands throughout the pancreas.

The pancreas is two organs in one

1. The exocrine cells of the pancreas secrete digestive enzymes into the duodenum.
2. The endocrine cells release two hormones, glucagon and insulin, into the blood.

Glucagon acts in exactly the opposite way to insulin. While both hormones govern the level of glucose in the bloodstream, glucagon is secreted in response to glucose deficiency. If there is an insufficient response from this hormone, the result is hypoglycemia.

Insulin is produced by the islets of Langerhans, which are specialized cells in the pancreas. Insulin passes into the general circulation and controls carbohydrate metabolism. Insulin regulates the utilization of glucose in the body. All body tissues, except the brain, require insulin for the absorption of glucose. If the pancreas fails to produce insulin, or secretes it in insufficient quantities, the result is a serious disease called diabetes mellitus.

A duct running the length of the organ collects pancreatic juice and passes it to the duodenum at the same point the common bile duct passes in bile.

During the process of digestion, the larger particles of protein, carbohydrates and fats, must be reduced in size and converted into simpler substances. This enables them to be absorbed through the walls of the digestive tract and into the bloodstream. Proteins are converted to peptones and polypeptides, which are then converted into amino acids.

Similarly, carbohydrates must be reduced. The large particles, starches or polysaccharides, are reduced to disaccharides, which in turn are reduced to monosaccharides. Fats are split into their component parts, fatty acids and glycerin. It should be noted that, with one or two exceptions, there is no absorption of food elements until they reach the intestine where fatty acids and glycerin pass into the lacteals of the villi, and amino acids into the capillary blood vessels. Fatty products are conveyed into the lymphatic system, entering the systemic circulation via the thoracic duct. Amino acids and simple sugars are carried by the portal veins to the liver.

This information will give you a good overview of how your digestive system works, and just remember, "chew your food" and "don't fake it out with gum or candy!"

A SHORT OVERVIEW: DIGESTIVE TRACT
Mouth/teeth/tongue: acceptance and chewing of food
Stomach: production of gastric juices (hydrochloric acid, pepsin)
Liver: over 600 different functions. Main one for digestion is production of bile
Pancreas: secretion of enzymes (breaks down carbohydrates, proteins, fats)
Gallbladder: secretion of bile (emulsifies fats, lubricates intestines)
Small intestine: absorption of nutrients (foods, supplements)
Large intestine: re-absorption of liquids
Rectum and anus: elimination of wastes

Detoxification

Detoxification

Colonics are one way to detoxify, but there are other ways to speed the body's ability to have a healthy system. Here are some more ideas.

PREPARING YOURSELF FOR THIS PROCESS INVOLVES:
- Changing your eating habits
  - Eat organic meat, fresh fruits and vegetables, whole grains and drink plenty of water. Be aware of toxic and extra salty foods such as junk foods, sugar, alcohol, etc.
  - Introduce minerals, amino acids, and essential fatty acids into the body.
- Cleaning up your personal environment
- Look for toxic chemicals in aerosols, cleaners, dishwashing products, deodorizers, laundry soap, glass cleaners, garden pesticide products, paints, toilet cleaners, etc.
- Replace your toxic personal care products
  - Chemicals found in perfumes, shampoos, mouthwash, toothpaste, deodorants, make-up, etc.
- Baths and skin brushing.
- Kidney cleanse, lymph cleanse, liver cleanse, parasite and Candida cleanse.

FASTING

Any fast you try needs to be followed carefully. **Check with your doctor first.**

If you are going on any fast for more than one day, the most important part is when you are ready to eat solid foods again. You need re-introduce foods back into your system very slowly; a day or two of broth, then fruit, then grains, and lastly other types. It should take you two to three days to get your digestive system back on track.

THE MASTER CLEANSER (THE LEMONADE DIET)

Before using the Master Cleanser therapeutically, it is recommended to read the book 'The Master Cleanser', by Stanley Burroughs, to have complete instructions and obtain optimum results.

Regular fasting for 1-2 days a month on this drink is very cleansing and rejuvenating, and for major fasting try 10 days.

The Master Cleanser helps to:
- Purify the liver
- Dissolve and eliminate toxins and congestion that have formed in any part of the body
- Cleanse the kidneys and the digestive system
- Purify the glands and cells
- Eliminate unusable waste and hardened material in the joints and muscles
- Build a healthy blood stream
- Relieve pressure and irritation in the nerves, arteries and blood vessels
- Lose weight

Recommendation for your Master Cleanser Program:
The Master Cleanser drink has no fibre, so it is recommend to use an herbal laxative such as teas, oils, herbs or pills. Prune juice is also a natural laxative. This will help to remove the waste as it is being shed from the colon wall. Otherwise, the waste tends to stay in the body, leading to fatigue and other problems.

Recipe:
- 2 tablespoons lemon or lime juice (1/2 lemon)
- 1-2 tablespoons of pure grade B maple syrup
- 1/10th tablespoons cayenne pepper (red) or to taste (use a really little bit)
- 8-10 ounces of purified water (very warm to medium hot)
- Combine master cleanser ingredients and drink.

You may double the Master Cleanser recipe and fill a large thermos bottle and drink all day long.

Grade B maple syrup contains a large variety of minerals and vitamins.
- These include potassium, calcium, magnesium, manganese, iron, copper, phosphorus, sulfur, chlorine and silicon. Vitamin A, B1, B2, B6, C, nicotinic acid and pantothenic acid are also present.

Lemons are rich in vitamin C, and they are beneficial for building up a resistance against infection.
- They are low in calories and high in potassium, apart from other minerals. 100 grams of lemon gives only 57 kcal of energy, 0.9 grams of fat and have 1.7 grams of fibre. Lemon juice contains oil, which studies show is a great remedy for colds, obesity, constipation, oral diseases, throat disorders, fevers, cold, beauty aid, stomach problems, dehydration and diarrhea, and relieves rheumatism by stimulating the liver to expel toxins from the body

Cayenne has been used as medicine for centuries.
- Gastrointestinal tract, including stomach-aches, cramping pains and gas.
- Diseases of the circulatory system; it's still traditionally used in herbal medicine as a circulatory tonic.
- Rheumatic and arthritic pains. Rubbed on the skin it causes a counter-irritant effect. A counterirritant is something which causes irritation to the area to which it is applied. This makes it distract the nerves from the original irritation (such as joint pain in the case of arthritis).
- Sore throat. If gargled with water it can work as an effective treatment for sore throats.
- Styptic. Application of cayenne powder has traditionally been considered to have a powerful coagulating ability.

One time, when I was on the third day of the Master Cleanse, I was at work and all of a sudden I could smell the best dinner ever. I actually went into the lunchroom to find out what was cooking. There was no one there, and nothing was being cooked. I went out and could still smell it, so I went back in. I was sniffing around (I know that sounds stupid but it really did smell good) and it ended up being the garbage can. I am telling you, I understood from that point on how a homeless person could eat out of the garbage can. It smelt like a gourmet meal in there.

Other detoxification *(under advisement of your naturopath)*

Respiratory detoxification
Oxygen is responsible for clearing the blood of toxins and wastes. Removing unwanted toxins in your environment, combined with powerful breathing techniques, will help to improve your oxygen intake.
- Mucous and toxin release
- Breathing aromatics/cleansing oils (lime, peppermint, eucalyptus)
- Some herbal teas can remove excess mucous, decrease mucous viscosity and production by reducing inflammation, prevents the formation and release of histamine and histamine chemicals, enhances immune function, increases lung capacity, and stimulate bronchial receptors to cause some level of dilation
- Reduce mucous forming food, such as milk and dairy, eggs, sugar, salt, gluten-rich grains and starchy foods
- If your reactions are due to allergies, reduce exposure to chemicals, dust, or animals
- Natural cleansing promotes healthy mucous membranes and minimizes excess mucous production.

Lymph and skin detoxification
The lymphatic system provides us with our immune defences, filtering foreign substances and cell debris from blood and destroying them. Congestion in the lymphatic system means the whole body becomes toxic because the body's disposal system essentially fails.
- Lymphomyosot, a homeopathic therapy (avoid eating or using any mint products, since it will lower the effectiveness of this therapy)
- Herbs that support the skin and lymph
- Antioxidants
- Drink plenty of water
- Epsom salt bath and scrubs
- Skin brushing with a loofah
- Do not use any body lotions that are occlusive (sealing), you want the skin to take in oxygen and expel the waste

- Body wraps
- Baking soda baths
- Castor oil packs (used to help draw the toxins out of the abdominal area)
- Fatty acids
- Exfoliating
- Massage (European Lymph Drainage)
- Hormonal issues can affect the skin
- Food allergies
- Rebounder (bouncing stimulates the lymphatic system)
- Saunas or steam bath (pushing toxins out) *Do not stay in the sauna too long, as it has a drying effect*
- Use organic makeup
- Any form of exercise that makes you sweat gets toxins out of the body
- Work on your liver, because most skin conditions come from the liver
- Exercise and deep breathing keeps blood moving, stimulates central nervous system and flushes toxins; sweat out the toxins
- Emotional clearing gets rid of the negative thoughts that cause blemishes
- Mud baths

A great detoxifying bath is ½ cup of baking soda and ½ cup Epsom salts. Soak for 15-20 minutes, washing with soap of a natural fibre. Within minutes, the water becomes murky and takes out heavy metals such as mercury and aluminum.

KIDNEY AND BLADDER
The kidneys are the main filtering system in the body. The two kidneys excrete excess water and toxic waste in the form of urine. They are also responsible for maintaining the PH (acid/alkaline) balance in the blood.
- Drink More Water!
- Divide your weight by two, and drink that many ounces of water per day.
- Cranberry juice (pure unsweetened) Note: If experiencing a kidney infection cranberry may be irritating, consider using uva ursi.
- Juniper strengthens the urinary system and helps eliminate excess water.
- Herbs, such as juniper berries, uva ursi, hydrangea leaf, marshmallow root, gravel root, bearberry leaves, horsetail, dandelion leaf, vervain and lemongrass help to dissolve accumulations and soothe sensitive membranes.
- The urinary system plays a huge role in detoxification by filtering the

blood of huge amounts of nitrogenous waste.
- Keeping the sweat glands open can also take stress off of the kidneys. In acute situations, causing a person to sweat in a sweat bath or sauna can cleanse the blood through the skin and generally relieve stress on the kidneys.
- Vitamin B6 and magnesium (take daily help to prevent oxalate stones from forming)
- You can dissolve kidney stones with several different herbs.
- Keep phosphate levels lower by being aware of high phosphate foods (e.g. meats, breads, cereals, pastas, and carbonated drinks)

DETOXIFICATION OF THE LIVER AND GALLBLADDER

The liver is the second largest organ in the human body, after the skin. The liver is the body's chief filter of toxins. Cleansing the liver and gallbladder of gallstones improves digestion. It is advisable to do a parasite cleanse before ridding the body of gallstones.
- Gallbladder flush
- Colonics
- Coffee enema. Caffeine in the coffee triggers the liver to dump toxins. Drinking coffee does not have the same effect, in fact, ingesting coffee causes the body to become acidic. Because of the negative effects of drinking coffee you need to drink two glasses of water for each cup of coffee you have
- Yellow dock extract affects liver function and enhances detoxification; sometimes used against arsenic poisoning.
- Milk thistle extract is a source of silymarin, supportive to the liver by reducing liver disease risks from solvents, paints and glues
- Red clover extract detoxifies the liver and gallbladder

EXTRA DETOXIFICATION NOTES:
- Activated charcoal binds intestinal toxins and unfriendly microbial growth
- Benzonite clay, a bulk laxative, binds toxins such as pesticides
- Psyllium fiber cleans the mucous lining of the intestines and increases the bulk of the stools
- Probiotics are a protective bacteria supplement
- Use herbs that support the digestive tract
- Candida cleanse (ridding the body of candida overgrowth is one of the most important things you can do for your intestinal tract. Candida can

create a host of unwanted systems such as headaches, fatigue, etc.)
- Parasite cleanse (parasitic infestations can be detrimental to your health, therefore it is important to address this problem)

CONTRAST SHOWERS
Contrast hydrotherapy, or water therapy, is the use of water (hot, cold, steam, or ice) to relieve discomfort and promote physical well-being.
- Hot water is chosen for its relaxing properties. It is also thought to stimulate the immune system.
- Warm (tepid) water can be used to relieve stress and reduce a fever.
- Cold water is selected to reduce inflammation.

Alternating hot and cold water can stimulate the circulatory system, improve the immune system, reduce inflammation in the joints, promote the removal of small molecules, and reduce the levels of lactic acid in muscles.

Types of use:
whirlpools, jacuzzis, hot tubs, pools and Hubbard tanks, baths, showers, moist compresses, steam treatments and saunas, plus internal hydrotherapy - colonic irrigation and douching.

EXTRA INFO
- Adding Epsom salts (magnesium sulfate) or Dead Sea salts to a bath is an excellent way to promote muscle relaxation and relief from rheumatism and arthritis
- Adding herbs and essential oils to water can enhance its therapeutic value.
- The Swedish are known to take a soak in a hot tub and then jump into the snow. The native Indians go into a sweat lodge and then jump into a creek or cold pool.
- Improving your metabolism will help improve your digestion and will aid in weight lose.

Try this procedure at home in the shower:
3 minutes of hot water, 1 minute of cold, alternating for approximately 12 minutes (you might have to start with less time to get your body used to the difference).

Tests to take

Did you know that you can have these tests taken by your doctor or naturopath?

ALLERGY TEST: WHAT ARE YOU ALLERGIC TO, AND TO WHAT DEGREE?
It was very interesting to go to the naturopath and have an allergy test done. Many naturopaths use what is called a Vega machine to test for allergies.

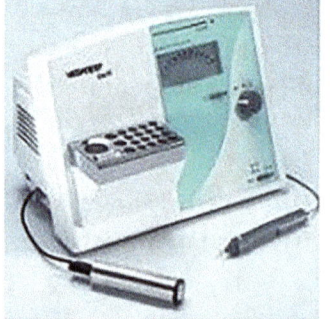

A Vega machine is a type of electro-acupuncture device used in Vega testing, which can diagnose allergies and other illnesses up to 70% accuracy. Helmut Schimmel modified the electro-acupuncture (developed by Reinholdt Voll in the 1950's) technique in the 1970s and presented it under the name 'Vega test'.

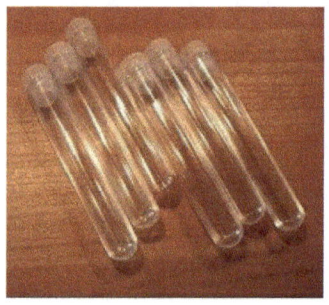

A small glass vial with product inside is tested: cigarettes, peanuts, grasses, wheat, chemicals, etc.
If you have read the information on Chinese body clock and muscle testing you will have read a bit of information on meridians.

Allergies are tested by placing the vial in a receptor, holding the metal rod, and having the practitioner probe your other hand with the electro-acupuncture tool. The Vega machine has a view panel which shows a needle or pendulum that moves up from zero depending on the reaction.

If you are neutral to the product the Vega machine does not move, if you have an imbalance with the vial (meaning your body does not like the product), the Vega machines needle moves. The higher it goes the worse the issue or allergy.

Blood Test

- Chem screen (blood chemistry)
- CBC (blood cell count)
- Ferritin (iron stores)
- Cholesterol
- TSH (thyroid)

Hair Analysis (Minerals)

- Taken from natural hair (not dyed)
- Sent into a lab to be examined (as hair grows out you can tell what is happening – 1/2" is about 1 month of growth)

Information this test can provide:
- Toxic elements: aluminum, antimony, arsenic, barium, bismuth, cadmium, lead, mercury, silver
- Nutritional minerals: boron, calcium, chromium, copper, iron, magnesium, manganese, molybdenum, phosphorus, potassium, sulfur, selenium, sodium, strontium, zinc
- Potentially toxic elements: palladium, thallium, tungsten, uranium, zirconium
- Other elements: cobalt, geranium, iodine, lithium, nickel, tin, vanadium
- Significant ratios: Ca:Mg, Fe:Cu, Na:K, Zn:Cu, Zn:Mn
- Interpretation of the result

Five pages of information are provided with this sheet. Green is good, while red is bad in either direction. Go to a naturopath for this test. One interesting thing, I noticed my cadmium was very high and into the red (under toxic elements); my husband and I had just finished painting the inside of our house.

Saliva test (pH – acid / alkaline)

Spit onto the stick and watch it turn colour, then match it to the pH range.

URINE TEST – SIMILAR TO THE SALIVA TEST, BUT YOUR URINE IS TESTED INSTEAD.

- Color – How dark or light the color is tells you how much water is in it.
- Clarity – Urine is normally clear. Bacteria, blood, sperm, crystals, or mucous can make urine look cloudy.
- Odour – Urine does not smell very strong, but has a slight "nutty" odor. Some diseases cause a change in the odour of urine. For example, an infection with E. coli bacteria can cause a bad odour, while diabetes or starvation can cause a sweet, fruity odour.
- Specific gravity – This checks the amount of substances in the urine. It also shows how well the kidneys balance the amount of water in urine. The higher the specific gravity, the more solid material is in the urine. When you drink a lot of fluid, your kidneys make urine with a high amount of water, which has a low specific gravity. When you do not drink fluids, your kidneys make urine with a small amount of water, which has a high specific gravity.
- pH – The pH is a measure of how acidic or alkaline (basic) the urine is. A urine pH of 4 is strongly acidic, 7 is neutral (neither acidic nor alkaline), and 9 is strongly alkaline. Sometimes the pH of urine is affected by certain treatments. For example, your doctor may instruct you on how to keep your urine either acidic or alkaline to prevent kidney stones from forming.
- Protein – protein is normally not found in the urine. Fever, hard exercise, pregnancy, and some diseases, especially kidney disease, may cause protein to be in the urine.
- Glucose – glucose is the type of sugar found in blood. Normally there is very little or no glucose in urine. When the blood sugar level is very high, as in uncontrolled diabetes, the sugar spills over into the urine. Glucose can also be found in urine when the kidneys are damaged or diseased.
- Nitrites – bacteria that cause a urinary tract infection (UTI) make an enzyme that changes urinary nitrates to nitrites. Nitrites in urine show a UTI is present.
- Leukocyte esterase (WBC esterase) – leukocyte esterase shows leukocytes (white blood cells [WBCs]) in the urine. WBCs in the urine may mean a UTI is present.
- Ketones – when fat is broken down for energy, the body makes substances called ketones (or ketone bodies). These are passed in the urine. Large amounts of ketones in the urine may mean a very serious condi-

tion, diabetic ketoacidosis, is present. A diet low in sugars and starches (carbohydrates), starvation, or severe vomiting may also cause ketones to be in the urine.
- Microscopic analysis – in this test, urine is spun in a special machine (centrifuge), so the solid materials (sediment) settle at the bottom. The sediment is spread on a slide and looked at under a microscope. Things that may be seen on the slide include:
- Red or white blood cells – blood cells are not found in urine normally. Inflammation, disease, or injury to the kidneys, ureters, bladder, or urethra can cause blood in urine. Strenuous exercise, such as running a marathon, can also cause blood in the urine. White blood cells may be a sign of infection or kidney disease.
- Casts – some types of kidney disease can cause plugs of material (called casts) to form in tiny tubes in the kidneys. The casts then get flushed out in the urine. Casts can be made of red or white blood cells, waxy or fatty substances, or protein. The type of cast in the urine can help show what type of kidney disease may be present.
- Crystals – healthy people often have only a few crystals in their urine. A large number of crystals, or certain types of crystals, may mean kidney stones are present or there is a problem with how the body is using food (metabolism).
- Bacteria, yeast cells, or parasites – there are no bacteria, yeast cells, or parasites in urine normally. If these are present, it can mean you have an infection.
- Squamous cells – the presence of squamous cells may mean that the sample is not as pure as it needs to be. These cells do not mean there is a medical problem, but your doctor may ask that you give another urine sample.

Nutritional Facts

A HEALTHY DIET WILL NEED:

- Carbohydrates – supply the body with energy
    - Simple – sugar (stevia is a good sugar substitute), grains, bread*, pasta*, noodles*

    *WILL NOT BE ABLE TO EAT ON THE ANGELIC FOODS DIET
    - Complex – vegetables and fruit

- Protein – growth and development
    - Meat (red/beef or wild game, white/fowl or pork, seafood/fish)
    - Eggs
    - Dairy products (cheese, yogurt, sour cream, milk)
    - Nuts (any)
    - Legumes (beans /peas)
    - Soy beans* you will not be able to eat tofu on the Angelic Foods diet, as it has been processed

- Fats – brain development, energy and support development
    - Monounsaturated fatty acids – 10 - 15 % of total calories (found in nuts and veggies, they reduce blood levels of LDL cholesterol without affecting HDL)
    - Polyunsaturated fatty acids – 20 - 25% of total calories (found in corn, safflower, sunflower, and certain fish oils, reducing blood levels of LDL cholesterol with affecting HDL. High in calories)
    - Saturated fatty acids – 10% or less of total calories (found in animal products, dairy, coconut oil, and palm/vegetable shortening. The liver uses saturated fats to manufacture cholesterol.)

- Micronutrients
    - Vitamins
    - Minerals

- Air
    - Oxygen – 21%
    - Nitrogen – 78%
    - Argon – 1%
    - Carbon dioxide
    - Water vapors

- Amino Acids
    - The building blocks that make up proteins (proteins are essential for life, needed for every living cell in the body)
    - Contain about 16% nitrogen

- Antioxidants
    - Are natural compounds that help protect the body from harmful free radicals
    - Free radicals destroy cells, impairing the immune system
    - Certain enzymes neutralize free radicals

- Enzymes
    - Essential for digesting food, stimulating the brain, providing cellular energy, and repairing tissues, organs and cells

- Water
    - Water makes up 70% of the adult body
    - Helps to detoxify the body of waste (dead cells, food, etc.)
    - Aids in digestion and helps keep your bowels regular
    - Lubricates joints
    - Improves cell function
    - Is an important solvent in the body
    - Water vapor in the lungs helps control oxygen concentration
    - Controls body temperature
    - Not enough water can cause fatigue and body aches
    - A minimum of 5 glasses is essential, but 8-10 glasses a day is great. Or your body weight divided by 2, then divided by 10
    - Caffeine/coffee depletes the body of water, so for every one cup of coffee you would need to drink two glasses of water
    - Caffeine free herbal tea and lemon water counts as a glass of water

***A person should drink water after all body treatments; massage, reflexology, etc., and also after exercising. Many people benefit from drinking room temperature water.

Do not:
- Use additives (used to lengthen shelf life, make food look appealing)
  - MSG
  - Artificial ingredients (aspartame – the body cannot metabolize)
- Overcook foods – this kills the nutrients. Barbequed foods can cause polycyclic aromatics hydrocarbons (dangerous carcinogenic /cancer causing) from the smoke of the drippings or if the food is burnt.
- Use aluminum or non stick cooking utensils (if this element goes into your system it can cause much damage)
- Use too much salt. Less than 500 milligrams of sodium a day is healthy (salt is needed to maintain normal fluid levels, healthy muscle function, and proper pH level of the blood) Processed foods (already made foods) have a high level of sodium (salt).

Calories
1000 calories or less is considered semi-starvation and the body slows down.

Female caloric needs to maintain body weight (men need approximately 500 calories more/day):
1. Number of inches over 5 feet multiplied by 5. (Example: If you are 5'8", you multiply 8 x 5 = 40)
2. Add 100. (40 +100 = 140)
3. Divide by 2.2. (140 / 2.2 = 63.6)
4. Multiply by kcals (kilocalories) for the amount of activity you have. (63.6 x 30 = 2000 calories)
- 20 - 25 kcals – inactive or sedentary (30 min or less / day) or to lose weight
- 25 - 30 kcals – moderately active (30 - 90 minutes of vigorous activity each day) or want to gain weight) or to maintain your weight
- 30 - 35 kcals – very active (90 minutes of vigorous activity each day) or want to gain weight)

A reduction of 3500 calories = 1 pound
1 to 2 pounds/week is healthy weight loss – this would equal 52 to 104 pounds in one year

OVERWEIGHT IS USUALLY CAUSED BY:
(Obesity is considered 25 pounds over your ideal weight)

- Genetics (horses are different – people are different; are you a mustang or a clydesdale – size, shape, speed, etc)
- Too many calories – what did you put into your mouth?
- Processed foods – no nutrients
- Fried foods – too much of the bad fat
- Emotions
- No planned meals
- Not enough exercise
- Digestive system malfunction
- Not chewing properly
- Liver and other organs not sending enzymes and other solutions to help break down food
- Chemicals
- Lymphatic sluggishness
- Endocrine system / Metabolism

THE AVERAGE DIET SHOULD CONTAIN:
- 35 - 45% fat
- 10 - 15% protein
- 40 - 45% carbohydrates

MEN

Height	Sm Frame	Med Frame	Lg Frame
5'2"	128-134	131-141	138-150
5'3"	130-136	133-143	140-153
5'4"	132-138	135-145	142-156
5'5"	134-140	137-148	144-160
5'6"	136-142	139-151	146-164
5'7"	138-145	142-154	149-168
5'8"	140-148	145-157	152-172
5'9"	142-151	148-160	155-176
5'10"	144-154	151-163	158-180

Height	Sm Frame	Med Frame	Lg Frame
5'11"	146-157	154-166	161-184
6'0"	149-160	157-170	164-188
6'1"	152-164	160-174	168-192
6'2"	155-168	164-178	172-197
6'3"	158-172	167-182	176-202
6'4"	162-176	171-187	181-207

WOMEN

Height	Sm Frame	Med Frame	Lg Frame
4'10"	102-111	109-121	118-131
4'11"	103-113	111-123	120-134
5'0"	104-115	113-126	122-137
5'1"	106-118	115-129	125-140
5'2"	108-121	118-132	128-143
5'3"	111-124	121-135	131-147
5'4"	114-127	124-138	134-151
5'5"	117-130	127-141	137-155
5'6"	120-133	130-144	140-159
5'7"	123-136	133-147	143-163
5'8"	126-139	136-150	146-167
5'9"	129-142	139-153	149-170
5'10"	132-145	142-156	152-173
5'11"	135-148	145-159	155-176
6'0"	138-151	148-162	158-179

Body Mass Index

Body Mass Index (BMI) is a number calculated from a person's weight and height. BMI provides a reliable indicator of body fat for most people, and is used to screen for weight categories that may lead to health problems.

Go to: http://www.cdc.gov/healthyweight/assessing/bmi/

Remember:
- Protein burns bad fat and builds cell life
- You need good fats (for brain function)
- Complex carbohydrates are needed for energy in the body (fruit and veggies)
- Simple carbohydrates create bad fat! (cookies, cakes, white bread, candy)
- Water cleans
- Laugh, live and love

These items can help in weight loss:
- Multi vitamin / mineral
  - Q10
  - B6
  - Zinc
  - Chromium
- Drinking a glass of water before you eat.
- Eating a bit of protein before any other food helps to balance your insulin.
- You need to heat up to burn off excess calories (imagine lard, hard to get off your fingers without really hot water and soap).
- Exercise to burn calories and gain more muscle.
- White fat is an insulating layer, just under skin (a little is good, a lot is not).
- Patchouli essential oil, pogostemon cablin, may cause loss of appetite.
  - Mix one or two drops into olive oil and apply a dab under your nose or on your tummy, one to three times per day.

When on a diet, there are many different opinions regarding what a person should eat. Here are a few examples:

Typical General Diet Guidelines (considered healthy for you)

- Avoid refined sugars, sweets or desserts. *too much sugar stops the T cells from doing their job
- Drinking a greens drink in the morning
- Drinking 1 tbsp of liquid chlorophyll daily
- Consider not having citrus fruits within 2 hours of a meal
- Drinking flaxseed oil (2 tbsp/day)
- Drinking carrot juice – 3 oz in the afternoon
- Drinking apple juice – 3 oz in the evening
- Drinking diluted prune juice daily
- Drinking a protein drink at least 3 times per week
- Eating ¼ of a ripe avocado at lunchtime each day
- Home juicing and drinking juice daily
- Drinking black cherry or concord grape juice daily
- Drinking 65oz of room temperature water daily (No more than 4 oz every half hour)
- Cutting down on acid and mucous forming foods
- Eating a reasonable portion of iodine rich foods each week
- Eating a reasonable portion of pyridoxine (B6) rich foods each week
- Deep breathing and exercises
- Sleeping with the head pointing north (allows new information in)
- Skin brushing
- 5 minutes of daily sunbathing for vitamin D
- Exercise (aerobic exercise can burn more calories, but is harder on the heart)

*T cells or white blood cells fight off infection by consuming the pathogen invader; viral, bacterial, fungal or parasite. Eating too much sugar will slow down or put the T cells to sleep for a while. This means the body will have no defence or ability to fight off the disease, and the invading pathogen can grow and mutate unhindered. Too much sugar for me is half a chocolate bar, I can feel my body slow down and it lasts about an hour.

CANADIAN FOOD GUIDE

http://www.hc-sc.gc.ca/fn-an/food-guide-aliment/index_e.html

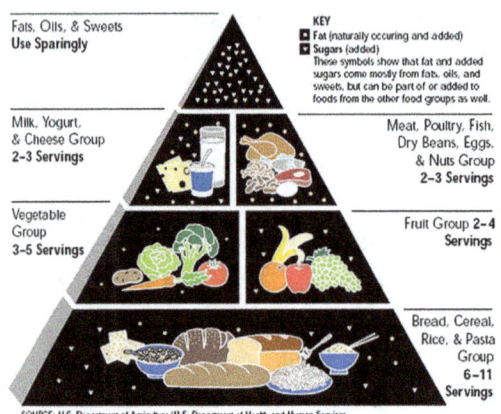

The Canadian Food Guide advises consumption from four food groups: grains, vegetables and fruit, milk products, and meat and alternatives. Any foods not accurately described by these food groups are termed "other", and are advised to be consumed in moderation.

For example, according to the Food Guide, a 35 year old women should aim to have these numbers of servings per day:
- 7 - 10 vegetables and fruit
- 7 - 12 grain products
- 3 milk or alternatives
- 3 meat or alternatives
- 30 - 45 ml (2 to 3 Tbsp) of unsaturated oils and fats

Depending on one's age and activity level, the aim is to consume a number of servings per food group that is high or low in the range provided. For example, male teenagers could aim for higher numbers, whereas elderly individuals could choose a number of servings that are lower.

FIBER

Natural fiber will not be absorbed into the body. It is a great broom, which naturally cleanses the colon.

I choose to use a juicer for my best results.

Set it up with a bowl under both the strainer and the tip.

Put the fruit or veggies in, they get chewed up by the metal teeth on the rotating grinder (just like what your teeth and stomach do), and juice will start to come out (this is the size of food particle that the small intestines can absorb into the body).

Eventually, fiber will come out the tip of the machine to be thrown away (I always find it amazing how long it takes before anything comes out). There will be a miniscule amount of nutrients left in the fiber coming out of a juicer. You will notice how similar the texture is to your feces, because that is what you're supposed to eliminate, fiber and dead cells.

If you are sick, it is better to use a juicer so you can better absorb the nutrients. If you are healthy, do not use this method as often because your body can do this for you.

Too much juicing isn't healthy. Do not juice and drink more than you can eat whole!

If you can eat only one orange at a sitting then do not juice more than one at a time. Also, watch how many beets you juice and drink; half of a small beet in a week is good. Beets are a very strong detoxification for the liver.

Remember, the body does need fiber, so juicing more than you should eat is not suggested.

For Your Health

Two major health issues
Sugar (diabetes) and cholesterol (high blood pressure/heart attack)

Following is a diet that helps to naturally change the results very quickly! Some people have positive results from their blood tests in as quick as one month.

Diet to control sugar and diabetes issues:

No
- Brown sugar
- White sugar
- Corn syrup
- Maplesugar
- Honey (a very, very little amount can be used)
- White bread or ground wheat products
- Dairy
- Pasta
- Alcohol
- Caffeine
- Refined/processed foods
- Carrots

Very important
- Do not skip meals
- Eat fiber with fruit

Slow down digestion
- Whole grains
- Barley
- Oats
- Rye
- Legumes

Good to eat
- Raw vegetables
- Raw fruits no more than 2 / day, eat with a protein
- Good fats
- Water
- Multi vitamin / mineral (chromium)
- Meat and eggs

Did you notice how similar the Angelic Foods diet is?

<u>Also</u>
- Reduce your stress with massage or meditation
- Exercise
- Eat smaller more frequent meals
- Make sure you are getting to your ideal weight

DIET TO CONTROL CHOLESTEROL ISSUES

No
- Meat
- Cheese
- Dairy
- Eggs
- Smoking
- Salt
- Sugar
- Peanut butter, most nuts
- Processed foods

Also
- Reduce your stress with massage or meditation
- Exercise
- Three meals daily

*Make sure you are at your ideal weight

Very important
- Lemon water
- Eat fiber with fruits
- Carbohydrates — up the fiber intake
  - Whole grains
  - Bran
  - Barley
  - Oats
  - Rye
  - Raw vegetables
  - Onions
  - Alfalfa sprouts
  - Raw fruits no more than 2 / day
  - Green apples
- Good fats (maximum 2 tablespoons / day)
  - Olive oil
  - Grapeseed oil
  - Flax
  - Many others
- Proteins

- Legumes (beans and lentils)
- Brazil nuts 2/day and almonds 5/day are best
- Soy products

Need
- Water
- Multi vitamin /mineral (Vit B Niacin, bee pollen)
- Green tea
- Psyllium
- Seeds (flax, pumpkin, sesame and sunflower)

Make sure to balance your protein intake with nuts and legumes! Great in a salad.

Ketosis (for losing weight)

Your body has three ways to burn energy
1. Carbohydrates
2. Protein
3. Stored body fat

BURNING BODY FAT IS KETOSIS?
Ketosis is a normal metabolic process, your body makes ketones. When your body doesn't have enough carbohydrates from food for your cells to burn energy, it can burn fat instead.

Many bodybuilders use this method to burn fat before a competition.

When caloric or carbohydrate intake is cut way back, your body can switch to ketosis for energy. Excessive exercise, pregnancy and uncontrolled diabetes can bring the body into ketosis (ketosis is a sign of not using enough insulin).

Ketones build up and can become dangerous when they lead to dehydration and change the chemical balance of your blood. Drink plenty of water!

You have to follow a customized diet, because you don't want the body to begin burning muscle for energy. The protein intake and muscle support, by way of mineral supplements, omega and multivitamins for the brain, is also important.

Less muscle means a lower metabolism, which means after the diet you will not have muscle to burn energy and you will crave more carbohydrates, which will store more fat and cause you to gain the weight back again.

Low-carb and Ketogenic Diets
You may know of the Atkins and Paleo diet.

Ideal Protein Weight Loss Method (www.idealprotein.com) is a great plan. Fast, safe and long lasting results! Yes, I have loved this body management system. Is it easy and worth every moment! I had results in the first week, and by week six I was down four belt notches and twenty pounds. The videos, coaching and variety of delicious protein foods were very beneficial.

The information the Ideal Protein's doctor gave about exercising to lose weight was fascinating. He stated that it is an excellent maintenance program, but food in the mouth is the only true cure to weight gain. Having your resting body in a high metabolic state is important. How many calories you burn when you are doing nothing or sleeping. The more slow twitch muscle burn or endurance you have, the better your resting metabolic rate will be. You will burn more calories at rest or during your sleep.

I found it interesting that when you do an aerobic exercise that brings your heart rate up, your body will automatically burn protein (muscle), which in turn will lower your metabolic rested state.

After you're finished with your weight loss, go to town and enjoy all the aerobic exercise you want. It will maintain your new weight and keep it off.

The Angelic Lifestyle will keep all that weight off. You might lose weight following the Angelic Lifestyle, but not as fast as the Ideal Protein Method, just saying... but I love using the Angelic Lifestyle to keep me healthy at my desired weight.

> "Your diet is a bank account.
> Good food choices are good investments." ~ Bethenny Frankel

> "Every single diet I ever fell off of was because of potatoes and gravy of some sort." ~ Dolly Parton

Natural Health Techniques

Muscle Testing

Muscle testing is a technique that has been used by healthcare professionals for many years, to evaluate the function and effectiveness of the muscles. Using muscle testing, we can ascertain which muscle is in a weakened condition, understand subconscious issues, and receive yes or no answers.

Body pendulum:
1. Stand upright.
2. Lean forward from the ankles saying ,"Forward is a 'yes', without falling" (you need to remain stiff, like a board).
3. Lean backwards from the ankles saying, "Backwards is a 'no', without falling."
4. Repeat this movement back and forth three times to program the mind.

Practice:
- Say, "My name is _____." If you go forward, that is correct.
- Then practice a fake name; if you go backwards, that is correct.
- Do a few silly, obvious questions to train your body. (e.g. "My shirt is _____.)
- Use vitamins; hold a vitamin (can be in the container) and ask, "Do I need to take any today?"
- If the answer is yes, then how many? For how many days? Add anything else you can think of. Try any other questions you can think of to train your body.

Note:
The mind is very literal. It will only answer literally what you asked. If you ask a bald man if he has hair on his head, I would bet his body will go forward. He may have eyebrows, a beard, a moustache, or hair in his ears/nose, etc. Literally, he does have hair on his head. If you asked him if he has hair on his scalp, then he would probably go backwards for a no.

If the body sways sideways, ask a different or more detailed question. If it stays still or does not move, it does not know the answer.

If the steps are not working, you are not responding with the body pendulum.
- Drink water
- Zip up three times (the ren/central meridian – the Touch for Health or Chinese medicine names – using your hand, pretend to zip up; start from the bottom of the body and follow up to the bottom lip).
- You might need to go to the washroom, or you may be in disbelief that your body is actually smart enough to answer you in the first place.

You may notice that professionals in muscle testing or kinesiology also use an arm technique instead of the body pendulum. I love to teach my clients the body pendulum so they can test themselves..

INTRODUCTION TO THE CHINESE BODY CLOCK (TIME OF DAY)

Chinese medicine uses meridians and tsubu points (specific areas on each meridian), which is the place the doctor would stick the acupuncture needle into.

Notice that there are two organs with the same time, one am and one pm.

The clock (time) shows you which organs are working and which ones are resting.

The Chinese call it high tide and low tide.
- High tide is when the organ is at its peak; when it is working.
- Low tide is a 12 hours difference; when it is resting.

Lung	3am - 5am
Large Intestine	5am - 7am
Stomach	7am - 9am
Spleen	9am - 11am
Heart	11am - 1pm
Small Intestine	1pm - 3pm
Bladder	3pm - 5pm
Kidney	5pm - 7pm
Pericardium	7pm - 9pm
Triple Warmer	9pm - 11pm
Gallbladder	11pm - 1am

Liver	1am - 3am

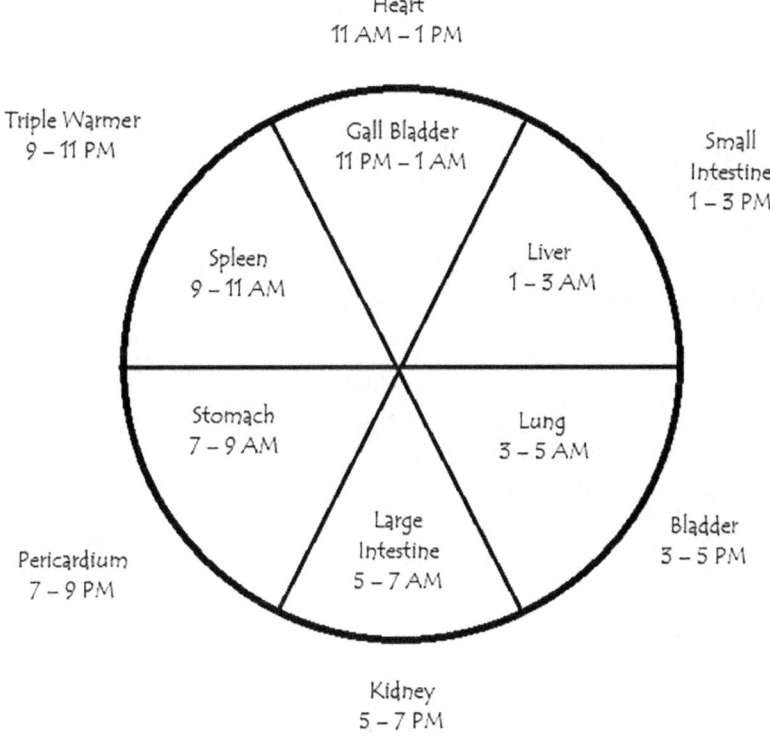

EXAMPLE:
- A client awakens to go to the bathroom (bowels) between 5am - 7pm (Large intestine) = high tide. This would also be the optimal time to treat and supplement the large intestine.
- This client may become fatigued between 5pm - 7 pm (opposite time, kidney) = low tide.

If you are having large intestine issues, it is advised to receive treatments and take supplements between 5am and 7am, as well as between 5pm and 7pm. This is not always convenient, but worth it.

To sum up the Chinese clock, any issues you are having with an organ, just look at a real clock and see what time it is. If it is in the same two hour period of the organ having issues, then this organ is already working its hardest, so do not do anything adverse to it at this time. If it's the opposite time, you should really not do anything adverse because it's at its weakest!

You can see why it's a known fact that many heart attacks occur in the middle of the night. Look at the clock!

Another interesting one, is if you wake up between 3 AM - 5 AM to go to pee, look at the clock... this is when the bladder is working the least. It cannot hold the urine any longer.

Once you have read the section on muscle testing/body pendulum, check to see if each meridian/organ is off balance. If any are off, then ask more questions
- Ask how many days, months or years it has been off
- Ask if you should go to the doctor about this organ
- Ask what foods you need to eat, or avoid, to balance this organ
- How long will it take to heal this organ?
- Do you need to take any vitamin supplements?
- How much water should you drink today?
- What exercise should you do today?
    - Any?
    - Walking
    - Running
    - Stretching
    - Etc.
- If you smoke, drink or do any drugs, should you quit? Now, or when?
- When is your Heavenly Day? Is it Day 42? If not, when?
- How long should you do this Angelic Foods diet? Forever? One Month, Three Months?
- Do you need to do any detoxifications? Which one?
- And anything else you can think of

Other Types of Sessions that will Benefit your Body

AROMATHERAPY

Aromatherapy is a relatively new term for the use of very specific plant extracts in healing. The practice or art of using such substances goes way back. When you study the history of essential oils, you follow a trail of use that leads to the modern term "aromatherapy".

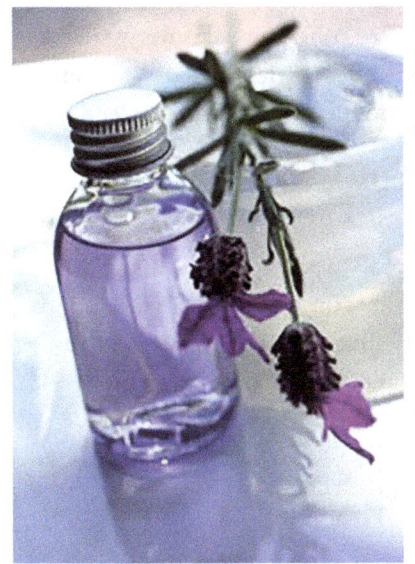

It is certain that the first to use plants as healing agents were the earliest men and women. Through experimentation, an oral history and knowledge of the different plants developed. As tribal culture matured and job specialization commenced, certain men and women would have honed a more detailed understanding of the healing and spiritual qualities of their local plants. In time, these "jobs" developed into the skills of shamans, spiritual leaders and healers.

There is evidence that the ancient Sumerians made use of scented herbs 4,000 years ago. The use of plants in their basic form as healing agents was clearly demonstrated when paintings on cave walls were discovered at "LA-SOO", in the Dordogne area of France. Carbon dating of cave samples has suggested that plants were used for healing as far back as 18,000 BC.

There are many essential oils that can promote aid to the digestive system. Just make sure you know the contraindications (what essential oils that can harm you) before using them.

Body Wrap

One of the better systems out there is the Universal Body Contour Wrap.

Universal Contour Wrap is the inch loss treatment that guarantees you'll lose at least 6 inches in just 2 hours, making it the perfect solution when you have to look your best for that special occasion.

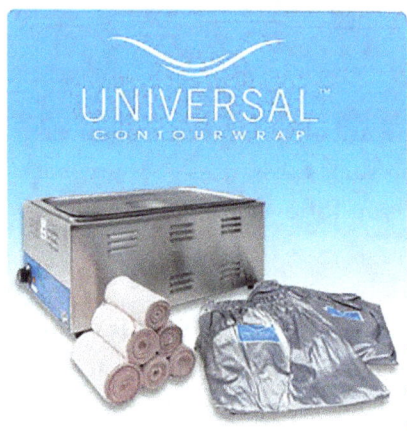

This wrap doesn't just deliver exceptional inch loss, but the unique clay formula and special wrapping techniques the therapists use also tighten and tone your body while exfoliating and cleansing the skin, so you will not only look great, you'll feel fabulous too.

There are other types of body wraps that help with detoxification and mineral or herbal absorption, such as seaweed or mud wraps.

You will be weighed and measured prior to the session. A specific mummifying technique is performed, and after you are slipped into a body suit you will lie down for approximately forty minutes. The practitioner will then remove the wrap, and you will wait (covered and laying down) for another fifteen minutes while the body dries. Then you will be re-measured to determine your inch loss. This session can be performed weekly until you have less than a six inch loss.

BODY SCRUB

A body polish is a spa treatment for the skin, like a facial for the body. A body polish session can be performed with any number of materials – salt, sugar, coffee grounds, rice bran, pecan hulls – and are usually mixed with some kind of massage oil and aromatic, like essential oils. If the polish uses salt, it might be called a salt scrub, salt glow or sea salt scrub. The exfoliation is usually followed by a shower (many spas do a dry application and remove with steamed towels) and an application of body lotion.

What happens during a body polish or scrub?

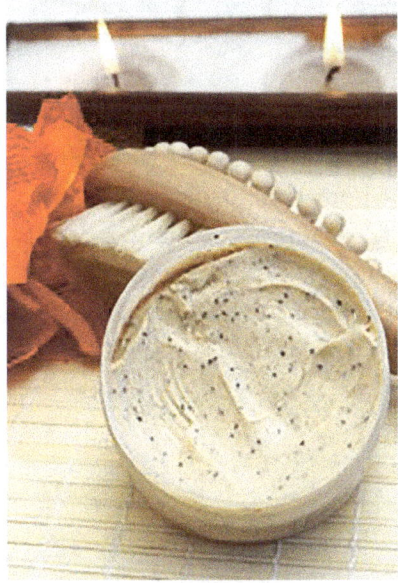

A body polish usually takes place in a room with a tile or linoleum floor. The practitioner may offer you disposable underwear, and will leave the room while you undress. You will start face down on a massage table covered with a towel, a sheet or a thin piece of plastic, or you may remain standing on a towel while the procedure takes place.

If performed while on a massage table, the practitioner will start by gently rubbing the scrub product on your back, the backs of your arms, and the backs of your legs and feet. You are draped with a towel or sheet, so only the part she is working on is exposed. Then you turn over, and she does the other side. Each area is cleansed with a warm steamed towel to remove the product.

Most body scrubs are combined with a massage.

BEAUTYTEK

The Beautytek system – Holistic face and body sculpting.

"Chinese medicine meets western computer technology with Beautytek treatments – the natural alternative to cosmetic surgery.

Now women and men can firm up and slim down effortlessly with Beautytek treatments. Previously only available at specialized treatment centers in Milan, Rome, London and Berlin, you can now experience the incomparable sensation of looking great and feeling energized with Beautytek at a facility near you.

During a treatment, the technologically advanced Beautytek computer uses gentle microcurrents to help boost cellular rejuvenation for a firmer, more youthful appearance. At certain points on the body similar to those used in acupuncture, a transfer of energy occurs, activating and enhancing the self-repair mechanisms of your body. The treatment removes toxins from the body, increases blood flow and lymphatic drainage." ~ Beautytek

See more remarkable results at www.beautytek.ca.

Beautytek applications
- Breast lifting and firming
- Body shaping and tissue tightening (neck, breast area, abdomen, arms, thighs, buttocks)
- Face contouring (double chin, jowls, eye puffiness)
- Fat and cellulite reduction
- Pregnancy stretch marks
- Acne and scars

Deep Breathing

Not only will deep breathing help you as a stress release technique, but the respiratory system is a very close partner to the cardiovascular system, providing oxygen to the body and removing carbon dioxide and other waste products.

Functions

The respiratory system is responsible for the following specific functions:
- Oxygen-carbon dioxide exchange via inspiration and expiration
- Speech production
- Maintaining proper pH in the blood

European Lymph Drainage Massage

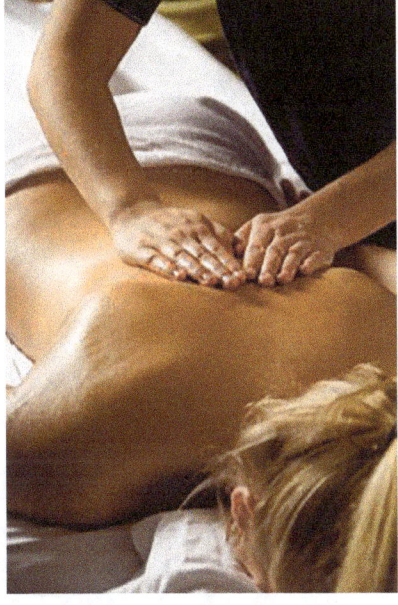

The benefits outlined below may not all be gained by the massage taught to practitioners. The approach to massage takes in the emotional and mental as much as the physical, and the benefits reflect these aspects. The body is worked with approximately two pounds of pressure.

The benefits of massage can be broken down into several categories. These are:
- Mechanical
- Physiological
- Psychological

Mechanical effects of massage are the impact the massage has directly on the muscles, skin, lymph, and circulatory system. It includes:
- Movement of lymph
- Movement venous blood (deoxygenated blood)
- Release and expulsion of lung secretions
- Movement of edema
- Movement of the digestive tract

Physiological effects
- Increased blood and lymph flow
- Increased flow of nutrients
- Removal of waste
- Encouragement of the healing process
- Resolution of edema and hematoma
- Increased extensibility of connective tissue
- Pain relief
- Increased joint movement
- Facilitation of muscle activity
- Stimulation of autonomic functions
- Stimulation of visceral functions
- Removal of lung secretions
- Sexual arousal
- Promotion of local and general relaxation
- Reduction of stress responses

Psychological effects are less obvious; however the following have been identified as benefiting from massage:
- Physical relaxation
- Relief of anxiety and tension
- Stimulation of physical activity
- Pain relief
- General feeling of well being (wellness)
- Sexual arousal
- General faith in the laying on of hands

Reflexology

Reflexology is the study of activating reflex points, usually on the feet or hands, which correlate with specific parts in ten anatomical zones.

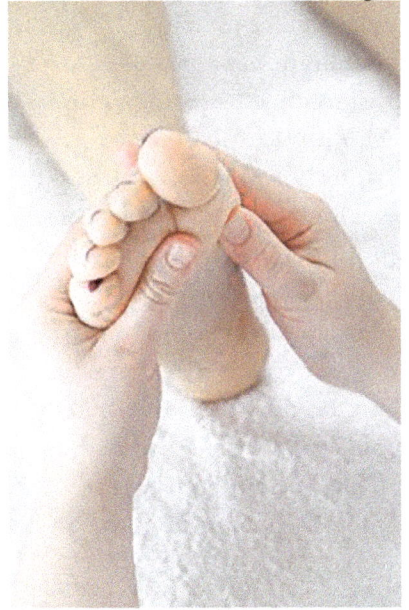

This practice of acupressure, energy and massage techniques stimulates the nervous system to awaken the autonomic nervous system and adjust the body to its optimum balance.

It is believed by some researchers that reflexology is actually a very ancient therapy reaching back to before 3,500 BC. It is thought that Buddhist monks brought the art of working the feet from India to China and Japan thousands of years ago.

Excellent technique for digestive system balancing, also for headaches!

Swedish massage

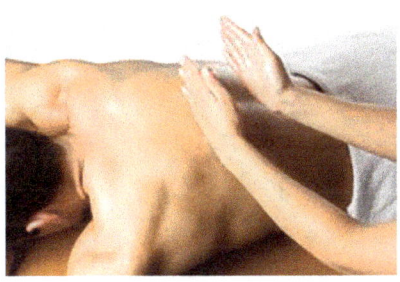

This type of massage is excellent for stressed or aching muscles. The muscles of the body are worked at approximately four pounds of pressure. Most Athletes use this type of massage to stimulate the body's system prior to a sports meet.

Many use this type of massage to relax after a hard week of work.

TABLE SHIATSU

The Japanese word Shiatsu is composed of "shi" meaning finger and "atsu" meaning pressure. The art of finger pressure applied on the acupressure meridians effectively releases muscular tension as well as toxicity.

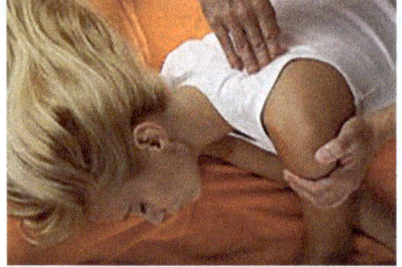

"Shiatsu therapy is a form of manipulation administered by the thumbs, fingers and palms, without the use of any instruments, mechanical or otherwise, to apply pressure to the human skin, correct internal malfunctioning, and promote and maintain health ..."

The pressure applied on certain points of the skin stimulates the body's natural curative powers. This direct pressure helps to release the excess lactic acid and carbon dioxide that contribute to muscular tensions. Shiatsu does not focus on any specific acupressure point, but a series of them along a meridian. These meridian lines are where the blood vessels, lymph, nerves and endocrine glands tend to concentrate or to branch.

The client is clothed and lying on a massage table.

There are many great natural health types of sessions you can choose from!

Your Emotions and Eating

Organs and the emotional meaning

Inside of Louise Hay's book, "Heal Your Body" (great book by the way) it tells about physical problems caused by emotional issues. Here is a peek.

Lung
- The ability to take in life

Colon
- Large intestine and small intestine
- Holding onto the past; fear of letting go

Stomach
- Digests ideas

Spleen
- Obsessions; being obsessed about things

Heart and pericardium
- Center of love and security

Bladder
- Anxiety, holding onto old ideas, fear of letting go, being peeved off

Kidney
- Criticism, disappointment, failure, shame, reacting like a little kid

Triple warmer - Glands
- Represent holding stations, self starting activity

Gallbladder
- Bitterness, hard thoughts, condemning, pride

Liver
- Seat of anger and primitive emotions

Meaning that you may be feeling this way and it is causing the related organ to have problems.

Ways to help you get over your negative eating habits

To purchase any of these sessions go to our website
www.constancesantego.ca

Emotional Clearing Technique or any type of counselling
The Emotional Clearing Technique is designed to find where in the person's body they are holding the issue and emotion (dis-ease), when the issue first began (origin), whose issue is it that's holding them back from success (emotionally, spiritually, mentally or physically), and how to release it.

This technique can pinpoint an exact moment in time when the client began creating the issue. It's beneficial to know the original point of the issue so that the brain (neurons) can release the negative emotions attached to it. Your memories are stored in the hypothalamus/limbic center of the brain, and will hold onto them forever unless told to remove them.

Patterns are created like a habit. A person repeats a situation over and over again, and the pattern or negative habit is created. Many holistic counsellors believe that this negative pattern is repeated for the person to learn a lesson and then move forward in life. Though, many people never learn the lesson and just keep reinforcing the negative emotion instead.

It is proven that we will act out the emotion we had when the original traumatic (negative) experience happened. This means you will act out the emotions of whatever age you were when it happened. Ever seen a fifty year old act like a ten year old? Funny when you think about how many people don't act their age when they are upset.
Example: Let's say at the age of forty-five, a similar situation brings back the trauma or bad feelings of when it originally happened at the age of four, our emotions and reactions would be like a four year old at any age until the person clears the emotional issue.

Big secret is... we cannot change others, we can only change ourselves. If a person does not like apple pie, it will never matter who made the apple pie, he/she will still not eat it. The emotion is embedded in the mind, and until the origin and truth of why they do not like apple pie is found, the person cannot change the feeling.

Hypnotherapy

Oxford definition of hypnosis: the induction of a state of consciousness in which a person apparently loses the power of voluntary action and is highly responsive to suggestion or direction. It's use in therapy, typically to recover suppressed memories or allow modifications of behavior, it has been revived but is still controversial.

Oxford definition of trance: a half conscious state characterized by an absence of response to external stimuli, typically as induced by hypnosis or entered by a medium.

Other Definitions:
"Trance is channeling magnetic forces to attain equilibrium of invisible magnetic body fluid" (animal magnetism) ~ Franz Mesmer

"Trance is a lucid sleep" ~ James Braid

"Hypnosis is a means of communication ideas; a means of asking people to accept ideas and examine them, to discover the intrinsic meanings, and then to decide whether or not to act upon those particular meanings." ~ Milton Erickson

"Hypnosis, or trance, is the means to quiet the conscious mind so we can access the subconscious and superconscious mind." ~ Connie Brummet

Excellent form of therapy to balance the emotional issues of your eating habits!

Reiki, energy balancing or chakra clearing

Reiki is one of the most ancient healing methods known to mankind. It originated in Tibet and was rediscovered in the nineteenth century by a Japanese monk, Dr. Mikao Usui. The tradition of Reiki is referred to in 2500 year old Sanskrit (the ancient Indian Language).

Any of the hands on approaches will help to balance the body, mind and soul!

Meditations

Mediations are a great way to have your conscious mind listen, while your subconscious mind changes and creates new pathways in your brain to achieve your desires.

Here is a meditation that you can have someone read to you, or go to my website www.angelic-foods.com and purchase the CD`s. When reading out loud, pause a few seconds when you see "… "

Angelic Foods Mediation Session 1

Get comfortable… really comfortable… not falling asleep… listening to my voice… enjoying what I have to say… very relaxed and very comfortable… any outside noises help you to relax even more… relaxing your whole body… knowing that my words will become your words… you can keep your eyes open or closed, whatever feels best… knowing you are safe and in control… ready to enjoy the Angelic Foods way of life…

Take a deep breath… in and out… Relax…

Take notice your feet… breathing… in and out… release and relax…imagine a cosmic garbage can if you like to throw your unwanted or needed energy into… Now notice your calves and thighs…… breathe… in and out… release and relax…and now your hips and torso…breathe… in and out… release and relax… your arms and hands…… breathe… in and out… release and relax… and last your neck and head…… breathe… in and out… release and relax…

Now that you are in a deep state of relaxation, not falling asleep, still able to hear my voice…just relax a few moments…enjoy this state of relaxation… You have begun this Angelic Foods healthy way of eating for your own personal reasons... maybe it is to achieve the slim and attractive body which you desire... maybe it is because your doctor told you to... or maybe you have allergies... or... maybe you just like to be healthy... I am going to give you some suggestions that will make this a permanent change in your living... these suggestions are going to take complete and thorough effect upon the deepest part of your subconscious mind... and will resonate in every cell of your being right down to your DNA... sealing themselves in the deepest part of your mind, body and soul... so they will remain there forever... becoming a permanent part of every cell of your brain and body... You may be surprised and amazed at just how effective these suggestions are going to be... and how much they will become a part of your everyday life... giving you brand new thoughts... brand new neuron pathways or patterns... a brand new method of action... these suggestions will make you a successful person...

If this is your first time listen to this, you will be learning a brand new method that you probably have never used before... if you have heard this mediation before and just love how it makes you feel... then absorb the benefits that suit you best... know that you have begun the positive approach for obtaining a healthy and attractive body which you desire... you have chosen this meditation as a positive means to attaining your goal... because meditation or trance is a great aid in permanently changing your emotional reactions to food and eating... you now realize that meditation is a positive new approach... a new positive approach to obtaining what you desire.

You will initiate a really good... positive... approach toward food and eating. As you initiate this good, positive attitude towards food... you will enjoy the taste of the healthy Angelic Foods... you will like the Angelic Foods... and you will easily eat the Angelic Foods... you will create a permanent positive change in your eating habits... from now on, you will prove to your own satisfaction that eating all your nutritious foods will entirely satisfy you... just like drinking all the water you need... you are going to work within the framework of your inborn normal reflexes... making a friend of your appetite... paying attention to it... for this is a good thing... healthy people have appetites... they pay attention to them... attractive people have appetites... they pay attention to them... meditation makes a friend of your appetite...

In the past, you've probably been paying attention only to half the signal from your appetite... namely, the signal that says, "Eat. I'm hungry." ...

but now you trust your appetite... you listen to all of what your appetite is advising... when it says "I'm hungry,"... you eat Angelic Foods... when the hunger feeling first disappears, and your appetite says, "I'm satisfied,"... you stop... you stop long before you're full... you are perfectly fed with nutritious foods that will stimulate your cells and regenerate your body, mind and soul... Angelic Foods taste sweeter and you love to chew the food you are eating... you love the feeling you get from the heavenly Angelic Foods...

Now, take three deep breaths and inhale all that is needed to make this permanent change to your subconscious and cells... to always choose these Angelic Foods... deep breath and exhale... exhale all the negative energy surrounding past emotions and memories that are not needed anymore... breathing in good energy... the Angelic Foods energy... breathing out any negative energy that may be holding you back... just put it into a cosmic garbage can... breathing in love light energy... all the love that you need... breathing out all that you do not... breathe in love... breathe out fear... breathing in the Angelic Foods energy all the way to your DNA... every cell nourished, beautiful and healthy...

...

Wonderful... knowing that every time you go into mediation, you will go faster, easier and deeper... now take another deep breath and wiggle your toes... coming back to the moment and opening your eyes... stretching... feeling alive, beautiful, successful and well... grateful for the Angelic Foods way of life...

What is your Carrot?

What carrot are you chasing?

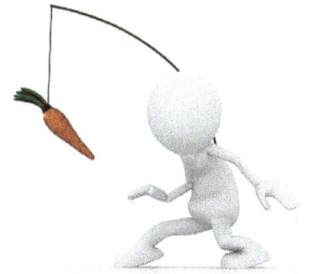 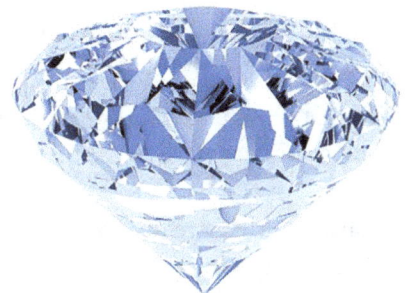

The carrot is what's keeping you on this Angelic Foods diet.

Most people need a goal or a reason to change old habits.
For me, the first time I tried this diet it was to gain the title "Grand Master", and every time I thought about going off the diet I would think about the title. I wanted the title more than the bread and sweets. As hard as it was, and trust me the urges and cravings were BIG, I was able to stick to the plan and do my 84 days.

The second time I did it was for my health. In the beginning, I still had many days that I second guessed why I was doing it, but writing this book helped to keep me going. I needed to succeed for my reader's sake. After a few months it was not for anything but the fact that I liked eating this way.

Whatever your goal or reason, it needs to be big or good enough to get you through the rough days. Something that you want, need or desire, more than the food! Be it weight loss, healthy eating, that new bathing suit, school reunion, yours or maybe your child's wedding, or to get a new boyfriend or girlfriend. I don't care what your carrot is, just find one. Try to make it a positive focus.

Remember pleasure and pain... pleasure will always win and you do not want the pleasure in this case to be breads or sweets. Find your carrot!!!

Your mind needs something to focus on that can be reasoned with, and can overpower the brain. If not, the brain will win those battles of craving.

TIPS FOR WHEN A CRAVING OR URGE COMES
- Drink some water, juice, tea (or coffee if you have to)
- Start to count
- Start to do something else
- Eat a carrot, piece of celery, raisins or nuts
- Start to cook lunch, dinner or supper

ANGELIC FOODS MEDIATION SESSION #2
Finding your carrot...

Get comfortable... really comfortable... not falling asleep... listening to my voice... enjoying what I have to say... very relaxed and very comfortable... any outside noises help you to relax even more... relaxing your whole body... knowing that my words will become your words... you can keep your eyes open or closed, whatever feels better... knowing you are safe and in control... ready to enjoy the Angelic Foods way of life...

Take a deep breath... in and release...

Take notice your feet... breathing... in and out... release and relax...imagine a cosmic garbage can if you like to throw your unwanted or needed energy into... now notice your calves and thighs... breathe... in and out... release and relax...and now your hips and torso...breathe... in and out... release and relax... your arms and hands... breathe... in and out... release and relax... and last your neck and head...... breathe... in and out... release and relax...

Now that you are in a deep state of relaxation, not falling asleep, still able to hear my voice... just relax a few moments... enjoy this state of relaxation... What is it that you can focus on when you need that extra help... when you are at family and friends for dinner... or really busy and do not have time to cook... what is that carrot that you can hold onto and lean on for support... Only you know what that carrot is... only you know how to get into your memories and unlock the carrot...

Take three more deep breaths... in and out...
in and out...
in and out...

Breath all the way down into your feet... sense your body... sense your soul... that's correct, I said soul... you can do it... you might feel it... see it... hear it or just know that it is there... but somehow you can sense your soul...

Your soul has all the knowledge of your memories you need... you need to know your carrot... what is strong enough to change your way of eating to the Angelic Food way of eating... forever... your carrot may be a word, sound, picture of an item or just an important thought or feeling... your carrot is very special...

You are now ready to unleash the knowledge... the secret... to your strength... the inner power you have to do anything you want... to achieve your desired goals, wishes and dreams...

Take a deep breath and imagine that you are on a path... this path can look, feel, sound or be any way you like... this path leads to your carrot... you will know when you get there, for as you turn a corner... there it is... your carrot... the thought, item, sound or feeling that is special to you...

...

Your carrot is impressive even to you... it has the power to overcome anything... now really sense your carrot and embrace its greatness...

Take a deep breath, and let all your cells of your body know that when you see, feel, hear or think this carrot... your special carrot... that it vibrates and creates the power you need to follow your truth of becoming and maintaining your health, body and mind...

Go ahead and try it... imagine your carrot... notice your body's sensations... how your body changes to adjust to the power needed... how wonderful it is... and every time you imagine your carrot it gets stronger and more powerful... giving you the energy you need to complete, achieve and maintain your goal...

Now let's really test it...

Imagine that in front of you is chocolate, bread or some other type of food that makes you unhealthy or weak... now take a deep breath... and bring your carrot; that feeling, sound, image or thought that your body gave you to use when you are being tempted...

There you go... notice how the temptation dissipates and goes away... how your carrot overcomes the sensation of the temptation and creates power to change and choose the Angelic Foods instead... notice how easy it is and how much easier it is every time you sense your carrot instead...

Let's try again...

Imagine chocolate, chips, pop... or whatever your thought went to... now take a deep breath and imagine your carrot... if you need to, imagine it glowing even bigger... radiating the power that you have... to choose the Angelic Foods instead... delicious meats, veggies, cheese, or fruit in any combination... that your body is nourished and happy, when eating this food... the Angelic Food... that it is so easy to say no and bypass the temptations...

You did great... and every time, when this food, Angelic Foods... you imagine your carrot, it is that much easier to have the soul's power... Wonderful... knowing that every time you go into mediation, you will go even faster, easier and deeper... now take another deep breath and wiggle your toes... coming back to the moment and opening your eyes... stretching... feeling alive, beautiful, successful and well... grateful for the Angelic Foods way of life... and carrot...

What if I Fail?

What if I Fail?

No, really... you think you failed. Did that mean you tried and it did not work? Or that you cheated?

I like what Wayne Gretzky once said, "You miss 100% of the shots you do not take." Well my answer would be to 'try, try, and try again'.

There have been days, when I am in a situation, that eating the foods that are not on the Angelic Foods Diet is just going to happen. It may be that I am at a friends or family members for dinner and it seems like the best choice is to just eat the food. Or when I have a heavenly day and it lasts for two days instead of just one.

I have decided that I like to eat the Angelic Foods way better, I feel better eating those foods. Really what I am finding is that the longer I eat the Angelic Foods way, the more I want to. I almost have to force myself to eat the other fatty foods, even the first bites don't taste good, but my mind thinks it does.

You have each and every day to try again. Just remember, it takes about three days to detox the food you just ate, so you might feel like you crave it for a few days later.

Try again... remember your carrot!

CHECK IN CASE THERE IS MORE TO IT
- Too many calories – What did you put into your mouth?
- Processed foods – no nutrients
- Fried foods – too much of the bad fat
- Emotions
- No planned meals
- Not enough exercise
- Digestive system malfunction
- Not chewing properly
- Liver and other organs not sending enzymes and other solutions to help break down food
- Chemicals
- Lymphatic sluggishness

- Endocrine system/metabolism

REMEMBER:
- Protein burns bad fat and builds cell life
- You need good fats (for brain function)
- Complex carbohydrates are needed for energy in the body (fruit and veggies)
- Simple carbohydrates create bad fat! (cookies, cakes, white bread, candy)
- Water cleans
- Laugh, live and love

The Important Role of Fitness

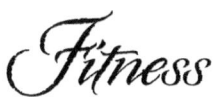

Fitness

The role of fitness *Remember to warm up before all exercise.
Exercise is an excellent tonic, which improves circulation, enhances digestion, strengthens the heart, tones the muscles, firms up the waistline, helps overcome constipation and improves your emotional and mental state of well being.

If possible, exercise in the open air, as oxygen is vital to every cell in your body. If overweight or in poor health, begin slowly and gradually increase your activity. Walking is a good beginning exercise.

Movement is essential. My saying is, "Move it or lose it". It's true for muscle tissue, joints and ligaments. Exercise every day for at least 10 minutes. When you are comfortable with the routine, increase your exercise to two 12 minute cycles each day. It can be a short walk around the block, walking up and down stairs, walking in the mall, or even deep full breathing at a fast pace for 10 minutes.

The body needs the essential oxygen that exercise brings. Make sure your iron level is proper. Iron is needed in the blood stream for the oxygen molecule to attach and be transported to all the systems in the body. Variety is the key to keeping your interest up. Movement oriented housework such as vacuuming, sweeping, dusting, washing floors, and washing windows are all excellent and productive forms of exercise. The keys to success are to find activities that you enjoy, that are accessible, and within your budget.

Start slow, beginning with 10 minutes the first day, gradually working up to 30 - 45 minutes per session. Remember, slow and steady wins the race!

SOME FORMS OF EXERCISE ARE:

Cross training
- Work towards 3 to 4 cardiovascular sessions of 20 - 60 minutes per week with 2 weight bearing sessions of 15 - 20 minutes per week. Flexibility and stretching exercises need to be practiced daily for a minimum of 10 minutes. Fitness is a discipline.

Weight bearing or strength training
- Vital to bone health and increasing muscle mass. Free weights or machines can be used at a gym or at home. Soup tins and other household items work well as weights. Elastic bands provide good resistance.

Cardiovascular training
- Benefits our heart and lung capacity, providing essential blood flow and oxygen throughout our bodies. Walking, swimming, cycling, rowing, jogging, hiking, dancing, and movement oriented housework are just a few examples.

Stretching/flexibility
- A daily session of full body movement, and rotations of the joints to limber up and awaken the body is recommended. Some of the many options include: yoga, Tai Chi, Qi Gong, 8 essential standing exercises, 5 Tibetan Rites...

Deep breathing
- Benefits are actually the same as cardiovascular training.

Team sports
- Fun, social and it helps with the COMMITMENT.

If you are going to run, here are some basics to know about first.
- Help protect yourself with socks. High performance socks will help keep your feet dry and comfortable by supporting and cushioning. A sock should be able to move moisture away from the foot. Blisters are caused from moist feet and friction.
- Stay away from 100% cotton socks. With a one hour run your feet can produce up to 250 ml (8 oz) of sweat. Cotton absorbs and sits next to your foot.

- Fit: Too big will bunch up and too tight will restrict toe movement.
- Should fit around the heel
- No toe seams
- Tighter weave in the middle of the foot (for support)
- Should fit your shoes (buy the socks and then your shoes)
- Shoes, not just any old runner!
- Most injuries are caused from the shoes support (or lack of it)

Shoe lingo:
- Heel counter – the most important part of the shoe. Support begins here. It is the thermoplastic molded cup that is hidden under the leather and cradles your heel for stability and proper stance.
- Midsole – the foam section found under your foot and above the outer sole. Used for shock absorption.
- Medial Support – a denser foam or plastic plug along the 'long arch' or the inside part of the midsole. This support guards from the shoe breaking down from excessive 'rolling in' during midstance (most important movement during walking or running).
- Outer sole – usually made of rubber, it is the bottom layer of the shoe. For traction and additional cushioning (differs depending on use).
- Toe box – the height and length of the toe box are critical for a proper fit. The toe box should provide enough room for the toes to spread and lengthen under high impact.
- Lacing system – mostly women have problems with heel slippage. Loop lacing technique and other lacing patterns can help with fitting and avoid irritation to certain areas of the foot.

Shoe types:
- Cross-trainers – cushioning of a running shoe with a bit of lateral support of a court shoe.
- Runner – high impact of heel to toe gait pattern for running or walking. Usually the lightest in weight, most cushioned and best ventilated. Great for problem feet.
- Court – limited cushioning, maximum support for lateral movements (bigger the court the better support you will need).
- Walking – less cushioning and ventilation. Looks nicer and more waterproof.
- Fitness – lighter than a cross-trainer, with better cushioning and flexibility. Softer 'indoor only' sole and increased lateral support.

- Orthotics – a customized, molded insole that often replaces the removable foot bed that comes in a shoe.
- Specialty shoes – water shoes, cleats, and dance shoes to name a few.

Fit
- When standing in a shoe, leave at least the width of your thumbnail between your longest toe and the end of the shoe. Runners or hiking boots may need even more room.
- The most important fit of the shoe is the heel to the ball of the foot. It should fit snugly but not uncomfortably tight. Leave lots of room in the toe box for the toes to spread when weight bearing.
- Consider your foot type. Does your foot pronate too much, or not enough? (Pronation will cause the sole of the foot to face more laterally than when standing in the anatomical position). Any pain?
- Different lacing techniques, adding a shim in the forefoot, or a heel sling may improve the fit in the heel.
- Did you get a bargain? Only if the shoe fits!!!

THE CORRECT BRA FOR WOMEN

Running or jumping can accelerate permanent stretching of the skin and sagging.

A great bra gives enough support, feels comfortable, doesn't chafe around armholes or rib cage, straps do not dig in, and the band beneath the breast shouldn't bind or abrade. The bra should be able to wick moisture from your skin.

Tips
- Small and medium breast size women – purchase a compression type sport bra
- Large breast size women – purchase encapsulation sport bra
- Clasp your hands over your head, and if the elastic band of the bra moves up, it doesn't fit properly
- The bra should be at least 25% lycra for a comfortable horizontal stretch
- Try on several types, and do a few movements (jump up and down, run in place, etc.) to feel how the garment moves.
- Breathable fabrics
- No snaps, hooks or zippers
- No rough edges that might chafe your skin
- Hang to dry (machine drying destroys elasticity and support)

Clothing
- Wear lightweight, breathable shirts made from high-tech fabrics which should wick moisture.

Fabric	Dry wt (g)	Wet wt (g)	Increase (%)	Dry Time (hr)
Akwatek	135.2	210.2	56	2
Dri-F.I.T.	130.7	225.2	72	2
Nylon spandex	86.6	131.4	52	2
Ultrasensor	76.2	110.4	45	2
CoolMax®	50.1	108.4	116	2
Cotton	82.6	214.5	160	7
Blend	151.8	375.2	147	7

By Runner's World

A great running course should teach you about:
- Shoes
- Stretching
- Injury prevention
- Clothing (layers)
- Breathing
- Core training
- Hill training
- Hydration (water) and nutrition (before a run: power bar, banana, fruit or yogurt)
- Motivation
- Race recovery

Eight Essential Standing Exercises

Pa Tuan Chin (Chinese) Pal Dan Gum (Korean)
Great exercises to gain flexibility and increase blood flow

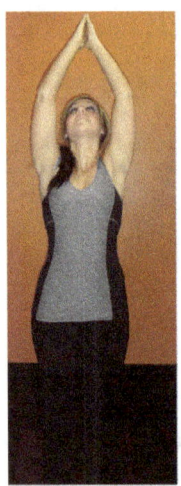

Upholding Heaven

Stand with your feet hip width apart, hands at your heart center. Interlace your fingers and raise your hands above your head. Gaze towards the sky as you stretch upwards. Exhale as you return your hands to your heart center.

Repeat 9 times.

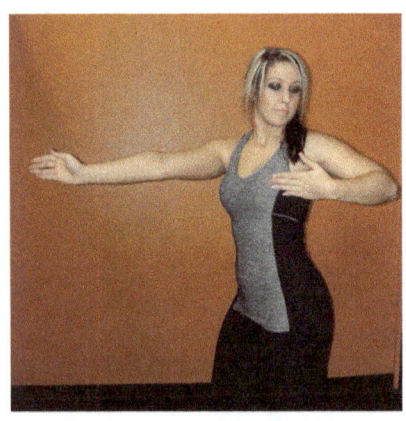

Opening the Bow

Stand with your feet hip width apart, arms at your sides. Turn to your right as you visualize that you are shooting an arrow. Draw back on your bow as you inhale. Release the arrow as you exhale. Return to center and continue this movement on the left side. Alternate sides.

Repeat 9 times.

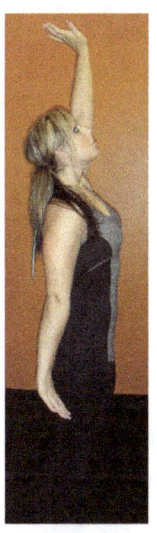

Reaching for Heaven and Earth

Stand with your feet hip width apart, hands at your heart center. Inhale as you raise your left hand above your head, palm facing upwards, with your fingers pointed inward towards the midline of your body. Simultaneously lower the right hand, palm facing down, towards the ground while pointing the fingers inwards. Exhale as you return your hands to your heart centre Alternate sides.

Repeat 9 times.

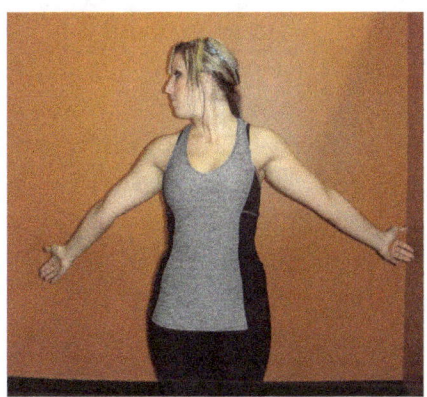

Looking Behind

Stand with your feet hip width apart, hands at your heart center. Inhale deeply as you open your arms to expose your heart center while you gaze over your right shoulder. Exhale as you return your hands to your heart center. Alternate sides.

Repeat 9 times.

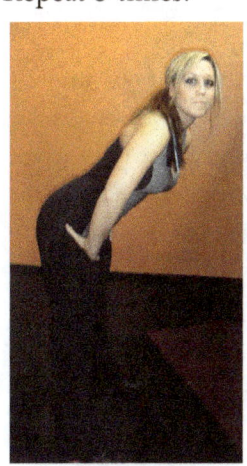

Wagging the Tail and Swaying the Head

Stand with your legs spread wide, feet more than hip width apart. Bend your knees. Place your hands above your knees. Begin to sway back and forth as you wag your tail. When you are comfortable with this movement begin to sway your head back and forth.

Repeat in the opposite direction.

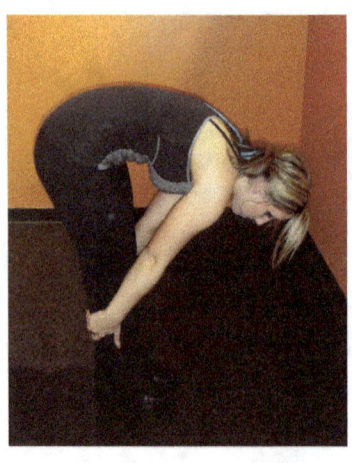

Pulling Up On the Legs

Stand with your feet hip width apart, arms at your sides. Exhale as you run your hands down the backs of your legs and hold onto your knees, calves or ankles. Inhale as you lift your heels up off the ground. Exhale as you return your heels to the ground.

Repeat 9 times.

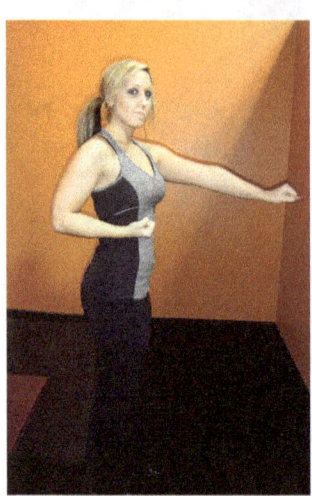

Clenching the Fists with Attentive Eyes

Stand with your feet hip width apart and your knees slightly bent. Make a fist with your palms facing up at waist level. Inhale as you open your eyes wide and smile. Exhale as you punch your fist diagonally in front while turning your fist over towards the ground. Inhale as you return your arm to your waist. Alternate sides.

Repeat 9 times.

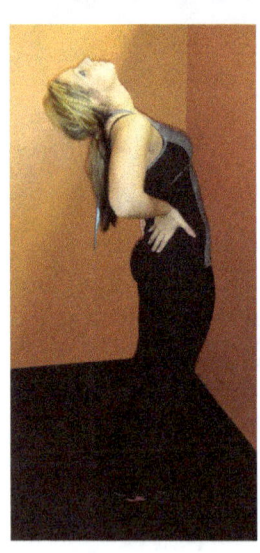

Stretching Backwards

Stand with your feet hip width apart and your knees slightly bent. Place your hands over your lower back with your fingers positioned downward. Inhale as you arch your back while gazing backwards. Exhale as you return to center. Repeat this movement 9 times.

Stretching forwards

Inhale as you raise your hand towards the sky. Exhale as you bend forwards from the hips reaching for your knees, ankles or toes. Repeat this movement 9 times.

*** REMEMBER TO BREATH***

<u>EASY EXERCISES TO DEVELOP YOUR CORE IN THE GYM OR AT HOME</u>

In 2005, I started to go to the gym and decided to hire a trainer. She was a wonderful and brilliant trainer. So different from any other that I had seen over the years. It used to be, when I went to a gym, the person in charge would set me up on the weights and tell me how many sets to do. I would almost not be able to walk the next day.

This trainer was different. She had me go on an elliptical machine for 10 minutes to warm up and then had me come over to an area where she assessed me by having me do what seemed like the simplest moves, until I tried them and could not do them. After about 20 minutes of trying all these exercises she informed me that my core, or stomach muscles, do not seem to be working at all. I was compensating using my quadriceps (thighs) and latissimus dorsi (upper back) muscle instead, which put a strain on my body.

She designed a few programs for me, but these are my favorite exercises:

20 minute warmup on a treadmill or elliptical
- Heart rate should be between 70% - 80% (127 - 146 bpm)
- If need be, start with 5 minutes and work your way up to 20

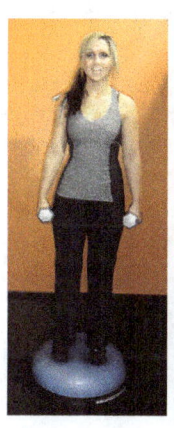 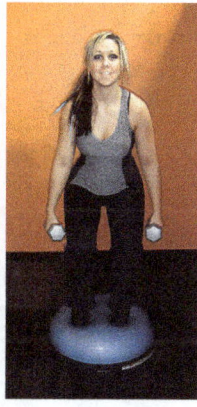

Sets: 1
Repetitions: 15
Load: 5 - 15 lbs weights
- Stand on the BOSU and do squats
- Think 'ABS tight' (tummy)
- Do a bicep curl at the same time as you squat
- Make sure your weight is evenly dis tributed

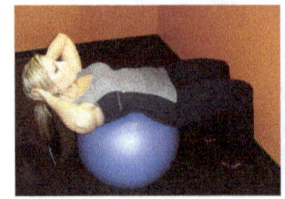 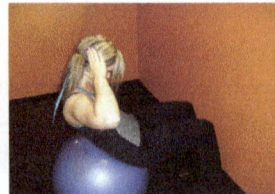

Sets: 1
Repetitions: 15
Load: body

- Feet against the wall
- Ball in the hollow area of your back
- Tuck in chin
- Pull ribs towards hips
	(you do not need to come all the way up)

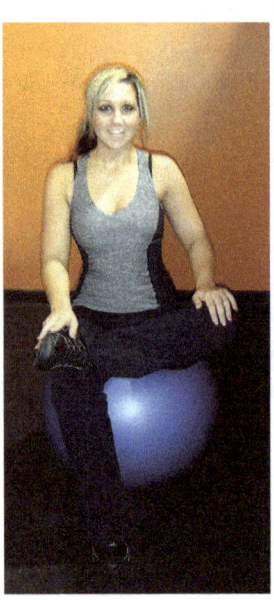

Sets: 1
Repetitions: 15
Load: arm
- Sit on ball
- One ankle over opposite knee
- Push lightly down with the hand on your bent knee
- Sit up straight and press knee towards floor
	(repeat on other knee)

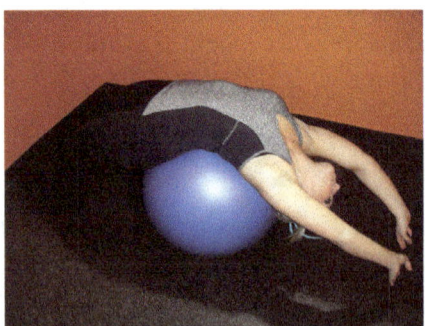

Total body stretch
- Do 5x

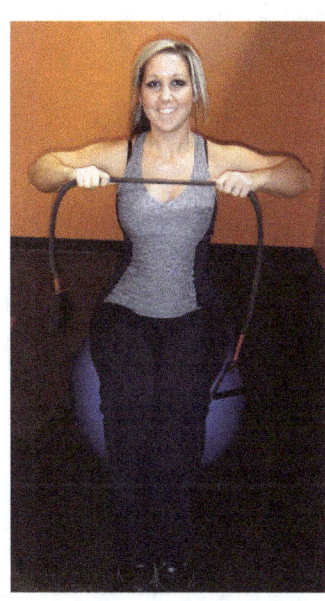

Sets: 1
Repetitions: 15
Load: Rd tube
- Using single elastic tube rope
- Sit on ball
- Focus is on the shoulder blades in your back
- Elbows parallel to the floor
- Squeeze the shoulder blades together
- Watch neck!

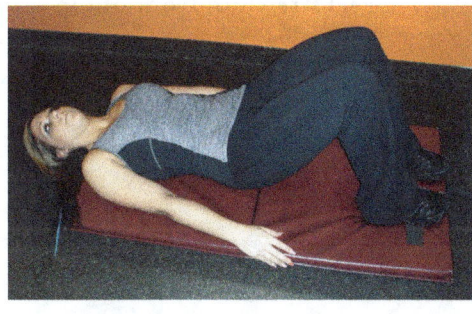

Sets: 1
Repetitions: 15
Load: 5 seconds

- Lay down on a mat with your knees bent
- Tighten abs but keep butt loose
- Keep feet in contact with the floor
- Keep shoulder blades down
- Try to isolate abs; pivot (slight lift - as if someone could slip a piece of paper under your bum)

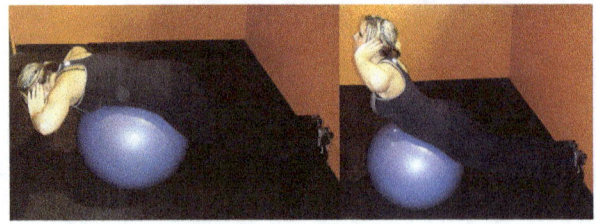

Sets: 1
Repetitions: 15
Load: body

- Feet against the wall
- Ball under pelvis
- Knees bent and off the floor
- Pull up until you feel tension in lower back

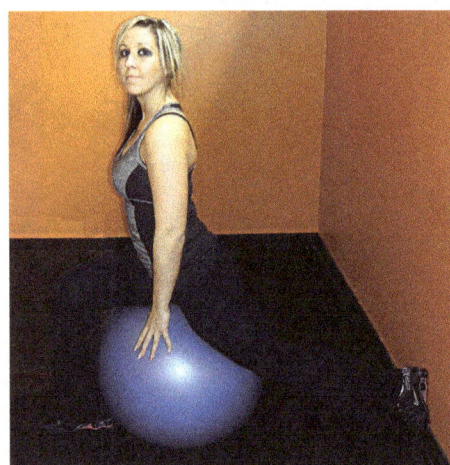

Sets: 1
Repetitions: 5
Load: Stretch each side
- Feel stretch in front of hip

and

Sets: 1
Repetitions: 5
Load: Stretch each side

- Hamstring stretch
- Sit on ball
- One knee bent, with opposite leg straight out
- bend forward - put weight on the knee - stretch (should feel stretch in straight leg)

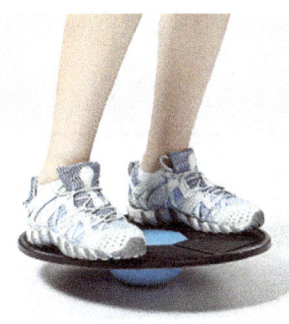

Sets: 1
Repetitions: 5 to 20
Load: body
- Excellent for core
- Stand on wobble or balance board (can use the wall at first)
- Even out your weight
- Objective is to balance for as long as possible

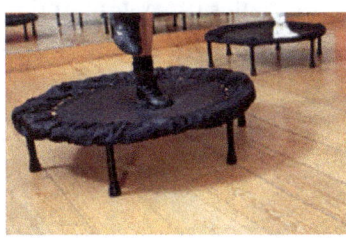

Sets: 1
Repetitions: 15
Load: body

- Excellent for lymphatic system
- Can use the back of a chair or wall for support if needed
- Lightly bounce on rebounder with one leg at a time, or you can bounce with both feet at a time

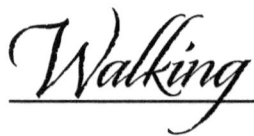
Walking

HEALTH BENEFITS OF WALKING
- Can be a great form of weight loss.
- Prevents physical disability in older people.
- Helps alleviate symptoms of depression.
- Walking strengthens your heart, improves your circulation system and helps to remove toxins.
- Is good for your brain. Significantly better cognitive function and less cognitive decline.
- Research shows that postmenopausal women who walk approximately one mile each day have higher whole body bone density.
- Just three times a week for 30 minutes can significantly increase cardio-respiratory fitness. Even walking 10 minutes a day will improve fitness!
- Helps to prevent Type 2 Diabetes. The Diabetes Prevention Program showed that walking 150 minutes per week (or 50 minutes 3x per week) and losing just 7% of your body weight (12-15 pounds) can reduce your risk of Diabetes by 58%.

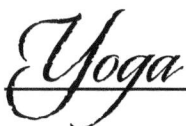

Yoga

Yoga is a physical, mental, and spiritual discipline, originating in ancient India. The goal of yoga, or of the person practicing yoga, is the attainment of a state of perfect spiritual insight and tranquility while meditating on the Hindu concept of divinity or Brahman. The word is associated with meditative practices in Hinduism, Jainism, and Buddhism.

Yoga has become one of the most common forms of exercise in North America; gentle yet effective to keep the body flexible and vibrant.

Glossary

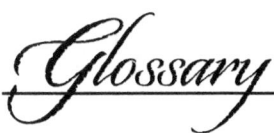

Glossary

TERMS FOR HERBAL PROPERTIES
- Analgesic – Relieves pain
- Antacid – Neutralizes excess acid
- Anthelmintic – An agent destructive to intestinal worms
- Anti-abortive – Inhibits abortive tendencies
- Antiasthmatic – Relieves asthmatic symptoms
- Antibiotic – Inhibits growth or destroys bacteria or amoebas. Some stimulate the body's own immune response
- Anticatarrhal – Prevents buildup of mucous in the respiratory tract
- Antidepressant – Uplifts, counteracts melancholy
- Antiemetic – Counteracts nausea, stops or reduces vomiting
- Anti-hidrotic – Prevents or increases perspiration
- Anti-inflammatory – Suppresses inflammation
- Antimicrobial – Reduces microbes
- Antipyretics – Cooling herbs. Reduce or prevent fevers
- Antirheumatic – Helps relieve rheumatism
- Antiseptic – Helps to prevent tissue degeneration and controls infections
- Antispasmodic – Relieves or prevents spasm
- Aperitif – Encourages appetite
- Aromatic – Having an agreeable odour
- Astringent – Contracts, tightens and binds tissues
- Bactericidal – Combats and destroys bacteria
- Bitter – A tonic made of ingredients with bitter flavours
- Carminative – Expulsion of gas from the intestines
- Cephalic – Stimulates and clears the mind
- Cordial – A tonic for the heart
- Diaphoretic – Induces perspiration
- Digestive – Aids digestion
- Diuretic – Increases urine flow
- Emetic – Induces vomiting
- Emmenagogue – Promotes and regulates menstrual flow

- Expectorant – Removes excess mucous from the bronchial tubes
- Febrifuge – That which cools and reduces high body temperature
- Fungicidal – Combats and destroys fungal infections
- Galactagogue – Increases secretion of milk
- Hepatic – Stimulates and aids the liver and gallbladder function. Related to the liver.
- Hemostatic – Arrest hemorrhaging
- Hypnotic – Induces sleep
- Hypotensive – Lowers blood pressure
- Laxative – A food, herbal or chemical substance which acts to loosen the bowels
- Lithotriptic – Dissolves and eliminates stones and gravel
- Narcotic – A drug which in moderate doses depresses the central nervous system, thus relieving pain and producing sleep but which in excessive doses cause unconsciousness, stupor, coma and possibly death
- Nervine – Reduces nervous disorders and response
- Nutrient – An agent having a nourishing effect
- Parasiticide – Kills or repels organisms living on or in a host organism
- Pectoral – Helpful for chest infections
- Rubefacient – An agent that reddens the skin by increasing blood flow to the skin
- Sedative – An agent which exerts a calming or tranquilizing effect
- Sialogogue – Induces the flow of saliva
- Spasmolytic – Arrests spasms or that which acts as an antispasmodic
- Stimulant – Any agent that temporarily increases functional activity
- Stomachic – Relieves gastric disorders
- Tonics – Herbs that promote the functions of the systems of the body. Give increased vigour to organs and nerves. Nourishing, rich in vitamins and minerals. Vulnerary – Prevents tissue degeneration and arrests bleeding in wounds

Bibliography

- Canadian Institute of Natural Health and Healing
  - Introduction to Anatomy/Physiology
  - Introduction to Herbology
  - Introduction to Fitness
  - Muscle Testing manual
  - Introduction to Nutrition
- About the Mind — Hypnotherapy and Meditation course manuals
- Heal Your Body: The Mental Causes for Physical Illness
  - Louise Hay
- Prescription for Nutritional Healing, 5th Edition: A Practical A-to-Z
  - Phyllis A. Balch CNC
- All licensed photos purchased through http://www.istockphoto.com/ca

About the Author

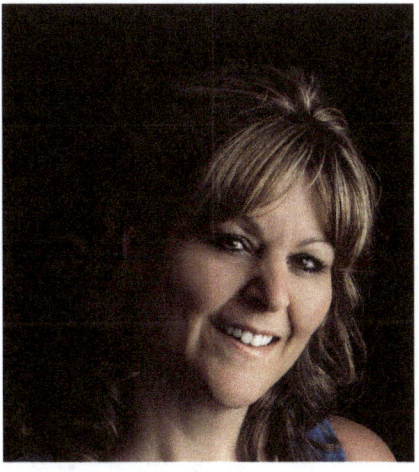

Constance Santego is a Canadian businesswoman, author, and artist.

Connie became world renowned from her Inspiration and Manifestation seminars and self help books: Intuitive Life, Fairy Tales Dreams and Reality, Your Persona Series, Angelic Lifestyle, and the Secrets of a Healer Series.

Her passion is teaching self-empowerment through the many ways to improve oneself; Emotionally, Spiritually, Mentally and Physically.

Constance Santego inspires you with many of her step-by-step workshops, books and seminars, taking you on a journey to transform your life and accelerate your path to achieving your dreams.

Angelic Lifestyle!
Enjoy your Journey, Constance

www.ingramcontent.com/pod-product-compliance
Lightning Source LLC
Chambersburg PA
CBHW070614300426
44113CB00010B/1521